Quick Start CD and Relaxation/Healing CD are inside the back cover.

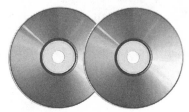

What People Are Saying about Prepare for Surgery, Heal Faster:

"This is the best book I have ever seen showing how to prepare for surgery — physically, emotionally and spiritually."

— Joan Borysenko, PhD
Author, Minding the Body, Mending the Mind
Co-founder, Mind/Body Clinic at Beth Israel Deaconess Medical Center
Harvard Medical School teaching hospital

"This book is essential reading for those who desire to participate in their healing. I enthusiastically recommend it."

— Susan L. Troyan, MD
Surgeon, Department of Breast Surgical Oncology
Brigham and Women's Hospital
Instructor in Surgery, Harvard Medical School

"This book is a great guide for anyone having surgery. It includes easy to follow steps that contribute to healing, self-knowledge and self-care."

— Jean Watson, PhD, RN, AHN-BC, FAAN
Distinguished Professor, Endowed Chair in Caring Science
University of Colorado Denver & Anschutz Medical Center
Founder, Watson Caring Science Institute

www.HealFaster.com

Prepare for Surgery, Heal Faster

A Guide of Mind-Body Techniques

Peggy Huddleston

Angel River Press
Cambridge, Massachusetts

This book is meant to be used in conjunction with your doctor. It is not intended as a substitute for medical advice. The reader should regularly consult a physician in matters relating to his or her health and particularly with respect to any symptoms that may require diagnosis or medical attention.

Published by Angel River Press
Cambridge, Massachusetts
www.HealFaster.com

Printed in the United States of America

10 9 8 7 6 5 4 3 2

Library of Congress Cataloging-in-Publication Data

Huddleston, Peggy
Prepare for surgery, heal faster: a guide of mind-body techniques / Peggy Huddleston – 4th edition
p.cm.

Includes bibliographical references and index.
ISBN 978-0-9645757-2-1 (alk. paper)
1. Surgery – Psychological aspects. 2. Holistic medicine
3. Mind and body. 4. Visualization – Therapeutic use. 1. Title

Cover watercolor of Exuma, Bahamas
"Clouds from Goat Cay"
By Jane Chermayeff

For Sam, my mother and those I love

You are a very important part of my dream
and my awakening.
And in those moments we touch heart to heart,
you are my vision and memory of oneness.

—Velvalee

Contents

Foreword

When I was in the middle of my obstetrics and gynecology residency in the late 1970s, spending hours on end every day in the operation room, I was inspired by Dr. Robert Mendelsohn's classic book, *Confessions of a Medical Heretic*.

The most memorable section was the chapter on "The Church in Modern Medicine" in which Mendelsohn described the operating room as a modern day *sanctum sanctorum* in which the ancient roles of the priests had been taken over by surgeons. He described the operation room as a place where elaborate rituals involving gowns, gloves and instruments were carried out in highly specialized and meticulous ways — with each surgeon, the equivalent of a high priest, having his, or occasionally her, peculiarities attended to in the process.

Mendelsohn's description, which I agreed with completely at the time, reminded me of something I was learning every day. The faith our culture used to place in God or the Divine has, to a great degree, been replaced by our collective faith in the powers of modern medicine to save and rescue us.

There is no question, especially in emergencies, that this power is of great benefit to all of us. And our cultural fascination with surgeons as saviors and rescuers is reflected in the most popular television shows of our times.

Since the operating room has become such apowerful symbol for curing in our collective imagination, why not take maximum advantage of this by consciously bringing your own innate healing ability into the operating room?

Peggy Huddleston and other pioneers in mind-body medicine understand that the full potential of the surgical experience can only be realized once the patient has become a complete partner in the healing process.

I often tell my patients that surgery, when properly prepared for, can become a healing ceremony that is both life-changing and life-enhancing.

This book is the most practical and complete manual for approaching surgery with maximal healing power that I have ever seen.

The only way to take full advantage of the healing through surgery is by acknowledging an ingredient that has been missing for far too long — the innate wisdom of the patient. All surgeons know that though we can perform operations well technically, we do not have the power to heal the tissue we have injured. This is up to the patients and their connection with their own inner wisdom.

Now imagine what would be possible if every patient openly and wholeheartedly embraced his or her part in the healing process — with the full cooperation and acknowledgment of their surgeon and anesthesiologist!

That is the direction in which Peggy Huddleston so skillfully points us — whether we participate as patients or surgeons. When we combine the healing power of the human spirit with the curing technology of surgery, we not only have the best of both worlds — we are also setting the stage for the miraculous to become commonplace.

Prepare for Surgery, Heal Faster and the healing guidance contained within it should be in the hands of everyone who is planning to have surgery. And though this book is specifically for those facing surgery, it contains much information that can be used by anyone, right now, for healing any illness, whether or not surgery is a part of that process.

This book should also be in the hands of all who perform, recommend, or in any way are connected with the process of surgery or healing.

I expect that in the next decade the guidance in this book will be given out to pre-operative patients as routinely as the operative consent form and the post-operative instructions.

Now sit back and relax. You're going to enjoy this journey into healing.

Christiane Northrup, M.D.
Past president of the
American Holistic Medical Association

Author of *Women's Bodies, Women's Wisdom*

Your Role
in the Healing Process

Love cures people, both the ones who
give it and the ones who receive it.

— Karl Menninger

This book shows you specific ways to enhance your
healing as you prepare for, and go through, any type
of minor or major surgery.

For some people, surgery is a simple matter of
having something fixed, removing a bone spur or a
benign cyst. If this is what you are facing, the mind-
body techniques you'll learn here will help you go
through routine surgery more easily and with greater
comfort. And you'll recover faster.

However, minor or major surgery can be frightening.
If you are afraid, the mind-body techniques will give

you ways to cope with your fears and actually feel peaceful during the hours, days and weeks before your operation. In turn, your calmness will improve your surgical outcome.

A review of the medical literature documents that people who prepare for an operation have less pain, fewer complications and recover sooner. This review was done at Harvard Medical School by Drs. Malcolm Rogers and Peter Reich.[1] Recent research studies are listed in the references.[2-15]

As a psychotherapist and a graduate of Harvard Divinity School, my clinical work, research and studies have focused on how people can use their emotions, attitudes and human spirits to enhance the healing process.

Over the past 18 years, I have taught workshops in self-healing techniques in Boston, New York, Philadelphia, London, Paris and Amsterdam.

Often in workshops someone will ask, "I am having surgery in a few weeks. What can I do to reduce my anxiety and make surgery less stressful? How can I have less pain and heal faster?"

In response, I developed five steps to prepare people for surgery. They give you specific ways to feel more in control at a time you can often feel helpless and vulnerable. They are easy to use and have no negative side effects.

Many people have told me how these techniques helped them cope with the emotional stress of surgery. And over and over, they have reported how amazed their doctors and nurses were at the ease and speed of their recovery.

Using these techniques will help you:
* **feel calmer before surgery**
* **use 23-50% less pain medication**
* **recover faster**
* **save money on medical bills.**

Research Study Documenting Benefits

For example in a study using *Prepare for Surgery, Heal Faster* with 56 patients having colorectal surgery, patients had significantly less anxiety before surgery, healed faster and were discharged from the hospital 1.6 days sooner than the control group. By the second day at home, patients used 60% less pain medication, had significantly less depression and insomnia and had a significant increase in patient satisfaction.

The study was done at The Lahey Clinic, a Tufts University School of Medicine teaching hospital in 2007.[16] The abstract is on page 247.

Five Steps to Prepare for Surgery

Step 1: Relax to Feel Peaceful

You will learn the skill of deep relaxation to reduce anxiety — and feel calm. Using the Relaxation CD designed to be used with this book, you will be guided through a process of relaxation. Feeling peaceful soothes your nervous system and strengthens your immune system. It also balances your endocrine and cardiovascular systems, creating the complex biochemistry that enhances overall healing.

Order my Relaxation CD or MP3 file at www.HealFaster.com or call 800 726-4173.

In addition, if you have any stress-related symptoms, such as tension headaches, migraines, insomnia, hypertension or anxiety, you'll find these symptoms diminishing or disappearing, depending on how well you master the technique of relaxation.

Research at Harvard Teaching Hospital

The benefits of my Relaxation CD were documented in a controlled study with 23 hospitalized patients not having surgery. Those who listened to the relaxation twice a day for 20 minutes for two days had a reduction in anxiety, used less medication for anxiety and had a significant, healthy decrease in heart rate. This study was done at Beth Israel Deaconess Medical Center, a Harvard Medical School teaching hospital.[17]

Once relaxed you'll learn to surround yourself with love as a way to promote healing. Ground-breaking medical research reveals what you may have always known: We all feel better when our hearts are filled with love — and we heal better too.

While research has shown that repeated experiences of frustration, anger and hostility accumulate in the body, suppressing the immune system and increasing heart disease, recent studies have documented that care, appreciation and love boost the immune system and enhance the functioning of the heart.

This innovative research has been conducted at the Institute of HeartMath in Boulder Creek, California. As individuals in the study focused on feelings of appreciation and love, there was a marked increase in their immune functioning, as measured by the antibody, salivary immunoglobulin A (IgA).

IgA protects the body against viruses and bacteria in the digestive and respiratory tracts. Individuals with higher levels of IgA are more resistant to colds and flu and have fewer respiratory infections.

When the same people experienced emotions of appreciation and love, their hearts reflected an increased ordering in heart rhythm patterns. Since the heart creates a large electrical field of energy that influences every cell, this has a very positive effect on the entire body.

By contrast, the individuals in the control group, who had not learned to focus on appreciation and love, had more chaotic heart rhythm patterns.[18-20]

Step 2: Visualize Your Healing
You'll learn to turn your worries into vivid, healing images. Using your intuitive knowing, the inner wisdom of your body will tell you what emotions and images will be most healing. As you use them daily to visualize your healing process, they will permeate your consciousness, facilitating your recovery.

Step 3: Organize a Support Group
You will learn a technique that allows the caring and loving thoughts of your friends and family to calm you during the half-hour before surgery.

Step 4: Use Healing Statements
You'll have less pain, fewer complications and heal faster if your doctor says three therapeutic statements to you during surgery. Medical research documents the dramatic benefits of the statements. It is your legal right to request them to be used.

The Healing Statements are on pages 259–263 which you give to your anesthesiologist, surgeon or nurse to say during your operation.

Step 5: Meet An Anesthesiologist
You'll learn to how benefit the most from your preoperative meeting with an anesthesiologist. You entrust your consciousness to this doctor. Yet people often do not meet an anesthesiologist until 30 minutes before surgery.

A research study at Harvard Medical School showed that arranging a meeting well before surgery significantly reduced patients' preoperative anxiety.[21]

In another Harvard study, patients having abdominal surgery used 50% less morphine and left the hospital 2.7 days sooner when their anesthesiologists instructed them in postoperative care. Patients in the control group never met an anesthesiologist and received no postoperative instruction.[22]

Even if your operation is tomorrow, you'll sleep better tonight if you call the Department of PreAdmissions and arrange a telephone meeting for today with an anesthesiologist. Having this doctor explain the procedures helps you feel calmer and more in control because you'll know what to expect.

Ideally, you will be reading this book one or two weeks before your operation. This will give you plenty of time to put all five steps to use well before surgery. The more steps you master, the better your results will be.

Quick Start

For a quick start, listen to my interview explaining my five steps to prepare for surgery. It is free to listen to or download at www.HealFaster.com. The interview comes with the Relaxation CD and MP3 files.

Only a Day Before Surgery

Even if you have only a day before surgery, you can dramatically influence your recovery by using these five steps. They are easy to implement.

After surgery, use Steps 1 and 2 to benefit your recuperation.

If you are motivated to do more, the epilogue shows how inner peace and love enhance your healing — physically, emotionally and spiritually.

Wake-Up Call

For some people, having an operation is a wake-up call — a call to look at their whole life to see what needs healing. It sets in motion a process that may require continued introspection for some time, before and after surgery.

If you hear this call — and answer it — it can lead to a renewed embrace with life.

For those who have made this journey, surgery became a doorway that opened to deeper meaning in their lives. At the time, they would never have imagined that it would become such an experience.

Preparing for Abdominal Surgery

Here is an example of how the five steps helped Elinor Elliot of Boston, Massachusetts. Elinor called me several weeks before having surgery to remove two ovarian cysts. She was agitated and fearful. Her mother had an occurrence of cancer and Elinor was afraid of the same thing.

To find what images would calm her, I asked, "When are you the most peaceful?" She said, "I love being in nature, seeing its beauty — feeling a sense of connection with the earth, trees and sky."

To reduce her anxiety, I guided Elinor through a process of deep relaxation. As she felt the tension letting go in her body, I asked her to remember a specific time she felt connected to the earth, trees and sky. Recalling it, she became calmer.

For her use at home, I gave her a CD of the relaxation process, like the one designed to be used with this book. With it, she could reduce her fear and feel calm. After listening to the CD, three times a day for a week, she began to feel in harmony with everything around her.

As If All of Spring Were Healing Her

It was spring, and she felt as if all of spring were healing her. The fragrance of the lilacs became healing, as did the singing of the birds and the warmth of the spring sun. She felt a resonance with all of life.

Her everyday world took on a new quality of peace. Because she listened to the CD so often, she could replay the relaxation process from memory, calming herself whenever she felt afraid.

In addition, she used techniques of visualization to picture the two cysts getting smaller. Three days before surgery an ultrasound test showed what is common with ovarian cysts — one of them had completely disappeared during her two weeks of preparation.

On the day of surgery at Beth Israel Deaconess Medical Center in Boston, she said, "I felt more peaceful than I have ever felt in my entire life as I lay on the gurney in the hallway waiting outside the operating room, listening to the Relaxation CD. As a nurse wheeled me into the operating room, my surgeon and nurses gathered around me, and I hugged them. It seemed like we were one team."

"As I went under the anesthesia, I heard my doctor say the positive statements that I had asked him to use. They worked so well that after surgery I needed little pain medication."

"My doctor commented that I was recovering much faster than three other women down the hall who had undergone the same operation. Of course, I was relieved knowing that the cyst was benign. I left the hospital one day earlier than planned. My two weeks of recovery were peaceful at home."

Peace

As you put the five steps into practice, you'll learn to let go of your fears about surgery and instead feel a deep peace. It will calm you before and during surgery and greatly enhance your healing.

It is an inner peace that most people have always known but have long forgotten how to find. For others, the peace goes far beyond anything they have ever known.

How to Speed Healing if
You Are Not Having Surgery

The book guides you through a healing process which you can use even if you are not having surgery. Read the entire book except for Steps 4 and 5 which refer specifically to surgery.

To enhance healing use the Relaxation CD. You'll find that relaxing helps you feel deeply peaceful. The epilogue shows you how to dwell in this peace for days and weeks. Doing so will speed your healing.

Prepare for Surgery, Heal Faster Training

If you would like to be trained and certified by me to give one-hour *Prepare for Surgery, Heal Faster Workshops*, I offer a two day training near Boston. You can take it in person or from your home.

It is for health care professionals and everyone else who wants to take it. Nurses and social workers get 13.5 CEUs. You will learn to give four one-hour workshops:

- Prepare for Surgery, Heal Faster Workshop™
- Reduce Anxiety and Cure Insomnia Workshop
- Lessen Chronic Pain Workshop
- Lessen Side-Effects of Chemo Workshop

These workshops are given in hospitals, HMOs, churches and corporations which self-insure.

For dates of trainings, see **www.HealFaster.com** and call my office at (800) 726-4173.

Practical Information about Surgery

> Whatever information helps make our situation more comprehensible is likely to contribute to our sense of control and a reduced risk of pain and illness.
>
> — Aaron Antonovsky

Before you put the five steps into practice, you'll want to spend some time talking to your surgeon about your operation. Prior to your meeting, write up a list of questions. Here are some suggestions of topics that may be important to you.

Feel Comfortable with Your Surgeon

The more confident you feel about your surgeon, the more it will help your healing process. A supportive doctor-patient relationship encourages you to get your questions answered and your emotional needs met. This allows you to relax, instead of feeling anxious or afraid.

As a result, you will feel calmer, creating the complex biochemistry that enhances healing.

Your calmness causes your parasympathetic nervous system to create a cascade of hormones that relaxes you. Your heart will beat at a more normal rate, your breathing will be regular and your muscles will relax.

These same hormones also strengthen your immune system. A healthy immune system defends your body against infection and helps you heal faster.

Conversely, anxiety and fear cause your sympathetic nervous system to be dominant, manufacturing the stress hormones that make your heart pound. Your breathing becomes fast and shallow, and you break out in a sweat. At the same time, these stress hormones actually suppress the functioning of your immune system.

As you can see, confidence in your surgeon is one of several factors that can influence a significant biochemical change in you. Of course you want a surgeon who is technically excellent, but don't underestimate the importance of having a good rapport with him or her.

If you have chosen a surgeon who is technically excellent, but one with whom you do not feel comfortable, ask your friends or a referring physician for the names of other surgeons. If you belong to a health insurance plan or an HMO, ask for the names of other surgeons within the plan. Continue to meet other surgeons until you find one who is equally competent, but with whom you also feel at ease.

Understand Your Coping Style

As you write up a list of questions to ask your surgeon, consider carefully how much you want to know. **For some people, too much detailed information creates anxiety; for others, too little is stressful.** Trust your feelings about how much information you need to feel well informed.

The amount of information that is right for you is determined by your coping style. Some people are "vigilant" types who cope best by gathering a lot of medical information. They like feeling in control, using their intellectual understanding as a way of maintaining that control.

If you are that kind of person, honor your way of coping and insist on getting all your questions answered. If you still have a nagging question after meeting your surgeon, don't hesitate to call him or her. By doing so, you'll feel better prepared and more comfortable before surgery, and as a result, you will have a better surgical outcome.

A very different way of coping is by "denying" or "avoiding." People with that type of coping style like to pull the covers over their head and go to sleep when confronted with a problem. They keep themselves extremely busy, as a way of not facing a situation. Their way of denying problems is an important means of self-protection and needs to be respected.

If that is your way of coping, tell your doctors so that they do not cause more stress by overloading you with too much medical information. Having to block out too many medical details will only create more tension.

Whatever your coping style, it's not likely to change. By understanding it, you can alert your doctors so that they can cooperate with it rather than unknowingly work against it.

Ask for Emotional Support

For your emotional support, bring along a good friend or a family member when you meet with your doctors. You also may want your friend to take notes or tape-record the meetings so that you'll have the information to go over later. That way you won't have the stress of trying to remember everything.

If your spouse or closest friend falls to pieces or has difficulty in medical situations, pick someone else who you know will be a comfort. Most people are up to the challenge of a health crisis, and as a result of going through it with you, you'll become even closer.

Small Hospitals Versus Teaching Hospitals

Small regional hospitals are fine for minor or major procedures, as long as your surgeon is board-certified. Teaching hospitals affiliated with medical schools in large cities also have well trained surgeons, who use the most up-to-date techniques and have access to state-of-the-art equipment.

If you are using a teaching hospital, usually you can request who performs the actual operation. Is it your surgeon, who is well known for his or her expertise and years of training or a resident just learning the ropes, practicing on your body?

In a teaching hospital, you'll be examined by many residents who usually have the time and enthusiasm to discuss your case. Of course, if you don't want to be poked and prodded by a stream of residents, you always have the right to say "No" to these examinations.

Regardless of what hospital you choose, ask your surgeon how many operations of this type he or she has performed. You may not want to be the third person to receive a new procedure.

Get a Second Opinion

Always get a second or even a third opinion if you feel the need. You don't have to worry that you will offend your doctor by getting other opinions. In fact, most surgeons will suggest that you get one, and most insurance companies will require it, although they will limit the number of opinions they will pay for.

If you belong to an HMO, you can always ask to consult with another physician within the health plan. If you want to see a specialist outside the plan, ask if your HMO will foot the bill. If not, you will have to pay for the second opinion, but it is often worth the consulting fee.

By getting opinions from other specialists, you can be sure that you are not jumping into unnecessary surgery. Sometimes another doctor may suggest a less invasive treatment and you can avoid surgery.

Medical Records

To save time, money and the hassle of going through the same diagnostic tests with different doctors, have copies of your medical records and test results under your arm when you see a new doctor. Since some doctors prefer to review your medical history in advance of your appointment, ask the consulting physicians when they would like the information. Hand delivering your records will avoid their getting lost in transit. For safety, always keep a back-up copy in your files.

Selecting Your Treatment

Be sure the treatment you choose feels right for you at a gut level. Be sure you believe in it. Your belief will make it even more effective.

If you are in denial about your diagnosis, doctor shopping and hearing other physicians' opinions may help break through your denial. In fact, seeing several doctors may assist you in becoming comfortable with your diagnosis.

But if you have an inner sense of knowing that doubts the diagnosis, continue to trust in yourself until your intuition is medically confirmed or denied — so that you feel no doubt about it. Doing this can be very challenging, especially when several medical authorities tell you a prognosis that goes against what you sense is true.

Always ask each doctor, "What are the different treatments for my condition? What are the most conservative and extreme types of treatment?"

For example, when a person has chronic back pain, an internist may suggest anti-inflammatory drugs to reduce the pain and muscle spasms, while a surgeon might suggest an operation. While both could be right from their points of view, you need to decide what is best for you. In fact, studies show that more than 75% of back problems heal without treatment in six weeks.

When you have a choice of treatments and the luxury of time, always consider the least invasive treatment first. It may be successful. If it doesn't work, you still have the option of other treatments, including possible surgery.

If time is of the essence because you have a condition that is worsening, you may not be able to wait and see whether the less invasive treatment proves successful. Even so, other opinions might offer you a better form of immediate treatment. Never take one doctor's opinion to be the final word, even if this doctor is considered an expert in the field.

This point is well illustrated by Dr. Isadore Rosenfeld. In his informative book, *Second Opinion: Your Comprehensive Guide to Treatment Alternatives*, he writes:

> The wife of one of my doctor friends developed severe headaches and attacks of double vision. She consulted a senior neurologist, who, after thorough testing, discovered a brain tumor. The patient asked for and was told the diagnosis. She was advised that surgery was not possible, and her only alternative was radiation which would shrink the tumor somewhat and alleviate the headaches, but would not cure her. This gallant lady settled her affairs and prepared to live out her last few months in the greatest possible comfort. Her husband, the doctor, knew better than to shop around for another opinion. This was, after all, an open-and-shut case confirmed by an eminent brain specialist.

But the patient was persuaded by a non-medical friend to see someone else. Reluctantly she consulted an equally prestigious neurosurgeon, who agreed with the diagnosis, but not with the treatment or outlook. He felt confident that the tumor could be completely removed.

With nothing to lose, my friend underwent surgery, and it was entirely successful. The tumor was a large one, pressing on her brain. After its removal, her symptoms disappeared and she returned to a normal life in a few weeks. That was 15 years ago.

Consent Form

Your surgeon is legally required to tell you the risks involved with your surgery so that you are fully informed when making the decision to have an operation. Your doctor will describe the risks and give them to you in writing, as a consent form for you to sign.

While it is important that you are fully aware of the risks, don't be frightened by the list of medical problems that have a one-in-a-million chance of actually happening. If you are highly suggestible, have a friend or spouse read the consent form to screen the information for you. Then sign it.

Your doctor has to inform you for two reasons. First, you need to know the risks involved when you agree to surgery. Second, doctors need to protect themselves from possible lawsuits. While the consent form protects your doctors, it may be damaging to your emotional state if you're given more medical problems to worry about. Find the balance for yourself, so that you are well informed, but not needlessly alarmed.

Arrange to sign the consent form as far in advance of the operation as possible so that you can avoid being confronted with a list of the risks half an hour before the operation. If it is emergency surgery, you obviously will have to sign it immediately before surgery. But with all other operations, ask to sign the form several weeks or at least a few days before surgery. This way you will have more time to process and release from your thoughts the negative possibilities written on it.

Date of Surgery

If you feel rushed into surgery, slow down the process by a week or two, if that gives you time to prepare yourself emotionally. Many surgeons have commented on how much better patients recover when they are truly ready. Don't get pushed into surgery too fast, unless it's an emergency.

Similarly, waiting too long can also be stressful. During a phone consultation with Jack Mommer, a grain farmer from Dike, Iowa, who was scheduled to undergo brain surgery at the Mayo Clinic in Rochester, Minnesota, Jack said, "These six weeks of waiting are killing me."

Even though it was medically safe to delay surgery because the tumor was slow-growing, the anxiety of waiting was not good for him. I encouraged Jack to call his surgeon. When he told his surgeon how anxious he felt and asked if the operation could be sooner, his doctor rescheduled the operation for the next week.

With this change, Jack felt greatly relieved and ready to get on with preparing for his operation and his road back to recovery — a recovery that astounded his medical team with its rapidity and ease. Clearly, Jack was ready.

As a curious aside, on Friday the 13th of any month, operating rooms are less busy because so many people are superstitious and avoid this date. When doctors need surgery, they pick Friday the 13th, knowing that they will get more attention from the hospital staff since operating rooms are less booked. If you are not superstitious, this might be just the choice for you.

Arrange for Patient-Controlled Analgesia

Ask your surgeon if patient-controlled analgesia (PCA) is available to use in your hospital room following surgery. A computerized device beside your bed lets you push a button to trigger a dose of pain medication if you have any discomfort or pain. You do not have to ring for a nurse and wait for a shot of medication.

Hooked up to the device by an intravenous line, you medicate yourself as you need it. This system lets you maintain a constant level of comfort. Research shows when people can regulate their pain medication, they use less of it, as compared to patients receiving intramuscular injections, the more traditional form of postoperative pain relief.

Programmed by your anesthesiologist, the PCA device prevents any chance of overdose, and the risk of addiction is minuscule: only 0.03%. In fact, the risk of addiction to any postoperative pain medication is equally minor.

Reducing and managing discomfort or pain has benefits beyond the immediate effect of feeling more comfortable. Studies show that pain suppresses your immune system. Therefore, the less you have the better your immune system can get on with your healing.

Your Own Blood for Transfusions

If you might need a transfusion during surgery, your own blood is the safest to receive. It's 100% compatible with your own. And there is no risk of being exposed to disease. The process that lets you use your own blood is called preoperative autologous blood donation. Units of blood can be drawn weeks before surgery and made available for transfusion as needed. For more information call the American Red Cross: (800) 552-0026.

Short-Term Psychotherapy for Anxiety

It is the most normal thing in the world to feel afraid and concerned about having surgery. But if you are extremely upset, the pending surgery may be triggering some other emotional issue. If this is happening, consider seeking short-term psychotherapy and use it as an opportunity to resolve this issue.

Releasing Emotions Promotes Healing

The more you can bring your anxieties to the surface and resolve them, the calmer you will feel before surgery and the better you will fare afterwards.

You might also talk about your anxieties with your surgeon or find a friend who will encourage you to discuss your feelings. As you begin to delve into them, you will probably encounter some repressed emotions. Give yourself permission to feel them. The more you experience them, at a level beyond words, the more easily they will be released.

If you resist feelings that seem irrational, they will persist. At one time in your life those feelings were rational, but you judged them to be irrational, refusing to experience them. Your ambivalence keeps them stuck, so that you half feel them and half resist them. As a result they never go away.

Embrace your emotions. Welcome them home like lost children. They are parts of yourself that you have rediscovered. Give in to them as soon as you can and work your way through them. You will feel more whole having done so.

Deep Emotional Release

The key to releasing emotions is having a therapist who encourages you to go into your feelings so that they can be discharged. An organic process takes over as your body involuntarily goes into a natural spasm of release. You may sob or even howl, discharging pent up grief or rage.

This is very different from "talk" therapy, traditional psychotherapy, although talking about emotions sometimes causes their release. To find hypnotherapists who can help you release emotions, see page 233 in the Resources .

For example, dealing with her extreme anxiety helped Bernice Lewiton of Waltham, Massachusetts, prepare for surgery. Bernice was scheduled to have a breast removed. As we talked, she cried.

Of course her crying was about the loss of her breast. But as we talked, she discovered she was also crying about an earlier loss, the death of her brother, who had been killed in World War II when she was 20. She realized she had never been allowed to grieve his death.

As Bernice talked about her brother, she cried and then stopped. As I saw her resisting her tears, I encouraged her to continue by saying, "It's wonderful you can cry. Let yourself feel how sad you are."

She looked at me, asking, "You mean it's all right to cry?" I said, "Yes, it's wonderful. Feel your sadness." She started to weep and then stopped.

As I encouraged her to cry, she began to sob uncontrollably. Bernice let go into that crying where you lose control and the crying just cries you.

After a while she said, "It feels good. I didn't know that it was all right to cry. When my brother was killed, we never saw our father cry. He kept all his emotions bottled up."

I explained that grieving was a process. But because we live in a death-denying society, Bernice had no way to grieve. By his example, her father had told her not to weep.

Bernice was like many of us who have within us, in the words of Dr. Elizabeth Kubler-Ross, "oceans of unshed tears." Because our society does not give us a time and a way to grieve, our tears are often suppressed.

Now that Bernice had allowed herself to open up to her emotions of loss, waves of grief would periodically return. Instead of avoiding her tears, she let herself cry, allowing the sadness to move through her and be released.

As her grief lessened, she came to understand that grief and loss were a part of life. By resolving her unfinished emotional business, she felt more settled before surgery.

Calmer before Surgery

If you are extremely anxious about a pending operation, dealing with your distress with the help of a good psychotherapist or friend will let you resolve it. As a result, you'll feel calmer before surgery which will improve your surgical outcome.

Summary

Practical Information about Surgery

1. Before meeting your surgeon, write up a list of questions. Take notepaper or a tape recorder to meetings with your doctors.

2. Be sure you feel confident about your surgeon. If not, ask a friend, a referring physician or your health insurance plan for names of other surgeons to meet.

3. Consider consulting another doctor for a second or third opinion. Ask what other treatments might be less invasive.

4. For emotional support, ask a good friend or family member to be with you during the meetings with your doctors.

5. Understand your coping style. Is it "vigilant" or "avoiding" and "denying"? Decide how much medical information you want to know.

6. Sign the consent form well in advance of your operation.

7. Be sure the date of surgery is right for you.

8. Ask your surgeon if patient-controlled analgesia (PCA) is available and appropriate for your use following surgery.

9. If you feel extremely anxious, consider short-term psychotherapy. Your pending operation may be triggering an unresolved emotional issue. Releasing it allows you to feel calmer before surgery, improving your surgical outcome.

10. Add your ideas here:

Step 1

Relax to Feel Peaceful

Peace is a condition of Spirit —
a part of that which we are,
existing in everything;
like the bones of the universe.

—Karen Goldman

Remember the last time you were deeply relaxed. Your body felt loose and comfortable, your mind peaceful. Maybe you were lying in the summer sun or listening to music or watching clouds drift across the sky. The situation — the warmth of the sun, the sweep of the music, the drifting clouds — caused you to let go of tension.

Now in preparing for surgery, you need to learn how to trigger this deep relaxation within yourself. Knowing how to relax, anywhere and anytime, is one of the best ways to cope with the stress of surgery. If you are mildly anxious or even very anxious, you'll be amazed at how easily you can learn to relax.

With a week or two of daily practice with the CD, you'll be so relaxed that you will feel peaceful in a noisy hospital hallway, waiting for your operation. And if you have a stressful medical test, you will be able to relax in the waiting room and during the test, making the process much easier.

Stress Causes 85% of Medical Problems

Research suggests that 85% of all medical problems are caused by stress. Stress-related symptoms range from tension headaches and migraines to lower-back pain, insomnia and hypertension.

When you are tense, you produce excess levels of stress hormones, such as cortisone and the catecholamines. Increased levels of these hormones diminish the activity of your immune system — your body's natural defense system against illness.

Higher levels of these chemicals reduce T-cells, natural killer cells, antibodies and other immune functions that protect you against disease.

Your immune system is controlled by your T-cells, or thymus cells, which originate in your thymus, a gland nestled between your breast bone and heart. Once T-cells identify foreign organisms, such as virus, bacteria, yeast or cancer, they stream to your spleen and lymph nodes to stimulate the production of other cells to fight the organisms.

Relaxation Strengthens the Immune System

While stress reduces the number of T-cells, relaxation can increase them. The interrelation between tension and lowered immunity was dramatically demonstrated in a study by Drs. Janice Kiecolt-Glaser and Ronald Glaser, psychologists at Ohio State University College of Medicine.

When they measured immune functions of medical students on the day of their examinations, researchers found decreases in the students' T-cell levels. After these same students were instructed in relaxation techniques, their T-cell counts increased. In fact, the more the students used the relaxation process, the greater the increase of their T-cells.[1]

Stress was first defined in the 1930s by Dr. Hans Selye.[2] When you feel threatened and afraid, your body shifts into a "fight-or-flight" response. Your heart beats faster, pumping more blood to your muscles which are tensed, ready to fight or run. A cascade of more than 30 hormones and neurotransmitters is released, giving you a burst of energy. At the same time, your blood sugar levels are elevated, while your immune system is suppressed and put on the back burner.

The fight-or-flight response is a natural protective reaction that can save your life in an emergency. It gives you energy to run out of a burning house or fight off an attacker. But having this response for days or weeks before surgery will exhaust you, suppress your immune system and lead to illness.

The hormones triggered by the fight-or-flight response are counterproductive before, during and after your operation. In this state of alarm, you feel frightened, anxious and constantly stressed. Mobilized to fight or flee, your skeletal muscles are chronically tense. During surgery, they need to be soft and relaxed instead of resistant to the surgical process.

Learning how to relax gives you a way to stop the fight-or-flight response. As a result, you'll be creating more of the hormones that relax your skeletal muscles, let your heart beat at a normal rate and help you feel peaceful.

This complex biochemistry of relaxation will allow you to go through surgery with a greater ease. It will enhance the functioning of your immune system, promoting a faster recovery.

Levels of Relaxation

There are different levels of relaxation. The first level is letting go of the physical tension in your body — the stress of a clenched jaw, tight shoulder muscles, a knot in your stomach or an overall sense of stress. You'll feel an enormous sense of relief as the tension eases up. The second level teaches you to let go of the specific emotions that are contributing to your stress.

Oneness

As you practice relaxing, you will find other, deeper levels of relaxation that can only be called sublimely peaceful. They are characterized by a feeling of connectedness or oneness. In nature, you may have felt connected or one with the whole landscape — the earth, trees and sky.

In the words of Willa Cather, the American novelist:

> That is happiness: to be dissolved into
> something complete and great.

Some people feel connected to something larger than themselves while listening to music or playing a musical instrument, when the music suddenly seems to play them. Others experience oneness through art or being with someone they love. Often women have a sense of unity during childbirth or while nursing their baby.

Tennis players call it being "in the zone." Suddenly, everything is smooth and flowing, and you can't miss. Others feel a sense of connectedness or flow while meditating, skiing or jogging. Runners often describe feeling "lighter than air, being able to run forever — almost like flying."

Many writers have described this state. The American novelist, Peter Matthiessen writes:

> The sun glints through the pines,
> and the heart is pierced in a moment of beauty.

Often people experience oneness when they become absorbed in what they see, becoming one with a flower or a mountain stream. In the words of the Zen Master, Huang Po:

> A perception, sudden as blinking, that subject and object are one, will lead to a deeply mysterious wordless understanding...

Transcendental or Transpersonal

Philosophers call this realm the "transcendental dimension" because you have transcended your everyday state of being and contacted the fundamental ground of being. It is also referred to as the "transpersonal dimension" meaning beyond the personal, beyond the ways you normally define yourself. In this state, you often feel more expanded and outside of a sense of time and space.

If this is your first experience with this dimension, you'll marvel at its gentle peacefulness. If it is a familiar realm, you can look forward to embracing it again. As you master going into deeper states of relaxation, you'll be learning to open doorways to a sense of interconnectedness and peace that is deeply healing.

As you use the relaxation process for several days or weeks, you will feel layers of tension releasing. You may experience the release as a gentle letting go. Sometimes you may feel your body shake or your muscles twitch as tensions dissolve. The sensation can be similar to what happens as you fall asleep. Your body slightly shudders or jerks, involuntarily. The shudder may last for a brief moment or go on for a few minutes. Enjoy it, knowing you are freeing pent-up tensions.

Releasing Emotions

Stress can also be released emotionally. For no apparent reason, you may feel a wave of sadness, fear, anger, hate, joy or gratitude move through you and dissolve, as you use the relaxation process. Let the emotions wash through you.

By welcoming each emotion, it will release more easily than if you resist it. Sometimes you'll recognize the events that the emotion relates to. Other times you will not. Either way is fine.

You may have experienced a similar release of emotion while having a massage. As the therapist's hands manipulate the deep tissues and muscles, buried emotions are spontaneously released. This same release is sometimes experienced during a session of acupuncture. A wave of emotion arises and subsides as it is discharged.

A few people experience tears when they begin relaxing. Some are tears of joy; others are tears of sadness. Welcome them as they move through you.

As you deeply relax, you are easing the wall of tension that holds back suppressed emotions, those emotions that once upon a time you swept under the rug to avoid feeling. In Western cultures, we have been taught and conditioned in endless ways to repress many "unacceptable emotions," such as anger, hate, fear, resentment, envy and sadness.

For example, remember a situation when you felt extremely angry and you could not express it. Maybe you were mad at your teacher, a boss or a friend. Those explosive feelings had to go somewhere. You had to clench your teeth, tighten your jaw or tense your shoulder muscles to hold it back. While that response may have been appropriate, it left you with a layer of muscular tension holding back the rage, and that rage remained lodged there.

Later in the day you may have released your fury by swimming, jogging or hitting a tennis ball. Or perhaps you went home and, unfortunately, blew up, taking it out on someone else. If not, that anger may still be stored in your body, along with a backlog of other emotions that you have suppressed over the years.

Burghild Nina Holzer, an American writer, poignantly describes emotions held in the landscape of her body. In her book, *A Walk Between Heaven and Earth*, her journal entry reads:

> Perhaps my womb wants to cry the story of the child I lost, of what wanted to be formed and what slipped out into darkness before it could be held securely by the arms near the heart.
>
> Maybe my throat wants to tell me of all the songs held back. Held back in fear, or in doubt, or in anger, all the songs that the heart already knows but that I have not voiced. Perhaps I need to walk in that place, down to my throat to the vocal cords.
>
> And maybe I need to write in my journal about the huge clump that sits there, blocking the air, blocking the sound, blocking the blood flow, causing pain. And maybe I need to discover that this big boulder sitting in my throat consists of a huge mass of words, compacted into stone — words pushed back, words too scary to face, words too tender, words too beautiful to admit. So many words wanting to be born, and all held back.

All It Takes Is Practice

As layers of tension and repressed emotions gradually release, it will become easier for you to let go into deeper levels of relaxation. All it takes is practice to develop the skill of relaxing.

However, it's not like getting a massage where you can lie still, letting somebody else do the work. In this process, you are the active ingredient. You do it. The more you are involved, the more relaxed you will become. With a week or two of daily practice with the CD, many people find that after listening to it, they feel even more relaxed than following a massage.

As you begin, you may easily experience a sense of peace. If not, the more you practice, the sooner you'll feel an inner peace. If there are two or more weeks before your operation, plan to use the Relaxation CD at least once or twice a day.

If you are experiencing a lot of emotional stress, insomnia and physical tension, use it two or three times a day. You can't overuse it. Go by how you feel, deciding how relaxed you want to be. As you practice, your stress-related symptoms will diminish or disappear.

Some people like to use the relaxation process when they wake up in the morning to center themselves and get their day off to a good start. Others use it in the middle or end of the day to let go of the stress that has built up during the day.

Choose one or two times of the day that are good for you to listen to it. Reserve these times for yourself. Write them in your daily schedule, if that will help you make the time to relax.

If you start canceling these appointments with yourself, pay attention to what you are deciding is more important, and find a time to reschedule your relaxation.

Support System

If it will encourage you, find a friend or family member who also wants to learn to relax. You can be a support system for each other. In person or by phone, check in daily, comparing your experiences with the CD. If your closest friend or spouse would like to learn, you'll have an added benefit. The more tranquil they become, the more peaceful you will feel around them.

If you don't have a friend or spouse who wants to learn to relax, at the very least ask a friend to be your support person.

Explain that you want to phone each day to say you used the CD. Tell your friend the key words you would love to hear each time you report in.

Knowing you've agreed to check in with someone may give you the extra nudge to use the CD on the days you might get too busy to take time to do it. Also, brainstorm with your friend about other ways to give yourself support for developing this new skill. Maybe you'll give yourself the treat of dinner at a favorite restaurant or a vacation in a place you've always dreamed of visiting.

To Begin

Find a quiet place where you will not be disturbed. If you are at home, turn on your answering machine. Turn off the bell on your phone or put a pillow over it. At first, minimizing distracting noises is helpful. Once you have learned to relax, you'll be able to do so with noise around you. That way, you will be calm even in a noisy hospital hallway.

If others are at home, tell them not to disturb you except for an emergency. Put a note on the door, saying, "Do not disturb until _____ ."
Listening to the CD takes about 25 minutes.

Choose a comfortable position, sitting or lying down. Stretch out on a bed or sit in a chair. You can alternate positions, learning to relax in any position. If you sit in a chair, be sure the back of your head is supported so you can completely let go. Loosen your clothing such as a belt or necktie so you can take easy, deep breaths. Do whatever you need to get very comfortable.

Use Headphones

At home, use any type of CD player you like. But at the hospital, you'll need one with headphones, preferably with an auto-reverse switch. Remember to take along several extra batteries as well as the recorder's electric cord.

Using the CD or iPod at the hospital will let you create your own private, healing atmosphere. Wherever you are, the headphones will block out distracting noises and give you privacy. Test the headphones at home to make certain they are working. Many people prefer to use headphones at home because they focus their attention.

If you get sleepy as you listen to the CD, gently bring your mind back to consciousness so you can follow the directed relaxation. However, if you continue drifting off to sleep, sit up while you use the CD, resting your head against a wall or the back of a chair. If you fall asleep in this position, your head will nod forward and wake you up. Bring yourself back to consciousness immediately so you can continue practicing.

You are learning an active technique. **You are the most important part of this process.** You need to stay focused on the CD so you can relax all the parts of your body.

The goal is to become deeply relaxed at a level of consciousness at which you would normally be asleep. In these deeper states of consciousness, you are highly suggestible, which allows you to influence your healing. But you have to stay awake to do this.

Relaxation Process

On the CD, you'll hear a background sound that helps you relax. It's made by two metronomes. One beats at the rate of a healthy heart, becoming slower as you relax. The second sound is soothing. Track 2 of the CD has no background sounds. You may like both or prefer one.

The CD begins, "Find a comfortable position and close your eyes. Take a deep breath and while exhaling feel a deep letting go." Taking a deep breath gets more oxygen into your bloodstream, making it easier for your nervous system to relax.

Then I'll say, "Focus your awareness on your neck. Release and relax and let go of any tension in this part of your body." Try this now. Put the book down for half a minute. Focus your whole attention on your neck, and feel a deep letting go.

You probably felt the muscles in your neck becoming softer. You may not have been aware of tension in your neck before you focused on it.

Imagine Tension Draining Away

Next you will relax your shoulders, arms and hands. As you relax your hands, I will ask you to imagine tension draining out through your fingertips. Then you will relax your chest, stomach, abdomen and back — the muscles and ligaments that go from the base of your neck all the way down to the small of your back.

Next you will relax your pelvis, hips and legs. I'll ask you playfully to imagine a door in the bottom of each foot. Picture opening the door and letting tension drain away. When the tension is gone, close the door.

Your Ideal Place

To help you enter a deeper, more relaxed state, imagine yourself in your ideal place of relaxation. It can be a real place or one you create in your imagination. For example, one woman imagines her favorite place from childhood: Lying in the warm spring sun, enclosed in a secret place in her family's garden. She smells the sweet honeysuckle and hears the birds singing around her.

Be sure the place you choose is completely serene and makes your whole body relax. A woman in my class in Paris said, "Why do my ankles feel so sore after this relaxation process?" I asked her, "What were you imagining as your ideal place?"

She answered, "I'm in Switzerland, skiing the last run of the day down the Wasserngrat, my favorite mountain in Gstaad. I tighten my ski boots before that run. Afterwards my ankles always feel sore."

I explained, "When you imagine your ideal place, you feel all your associations with that place." Just remembering skiing down the Wasserngrat brought back the soreness in her ankles, even though she was stretched out on a blanket in a meeting room in Paris.

You'll want all your associations and memories to be positive. If they are not, select a different place. The woman said, "I'll choose how I feel soaking in the sauna after a day of skiing. There all of me feels wonderful."

In Your Ideal Place
Imagine yourself <u>in</u> your ideal place rather than looking at a picture of yourself there. Feel the warmth of the sun on your body rather than seeing a picture of yourself lying in the sun. Experience all the sensations as if they are happening <u>now</u>.

Each time you use the relaxation process, the sights, sounds, smells and sensations of your ideal place will become more vivid. With practice, you'll be able to think of your place and, in a few moments, feel calm.

For instance, if you are sitting in a waiting room about to undergo some medical tests and you are tense, imagine yourself in your ideal place. If it's a favorite beach, feel the warmth of the sun, hear the waves breaking on the sand and smell the fresh sea air. As you relax, the tension will subside and you will be peaceful.

You also might use your CD player and headphones to guide you through the relaxation process while you wait for a test and while you undergo it.

Someone Easy to Love

Next the CD asks you to think of a person or pet who is easy to love. "Let your mind go back to a time you felt a great deal of love for and from the other. Feel these emotions now."

Don't settle for the "idea" of love. Instead recall a specific scene when you felt loved. Maybe it's how you feel now with your partner. If not, maybe it was the way your mother, father or grandmother hugged you as a child. Perhaps you felt a bonded connection with your dog or cat. As you remember it, you may experience a warm glow in your heart.

As you listen to the CD, recalling the love in that specific scene, the glow will get bigger. Let it fill your heart and surround you.

If you want to fill your heart faster, recall the love in the scene hundreds of times throughout the day. With practice, you'll be able to create that glow in your heart, having it spread through your chest.

You'll be learning how to center yourself in the love of your heart — instead of your mind. Years of western education have trained us to be centered in our minds, which has shifted us out of the love in our hearts.

Love Is Always There

Opening your heart will reconnect you to a larger field of love that surrounds us all. We live immersed in a palpable field of love, yet many don't feel it. Instead they experience an emptiness — the absence of love.

But the love they long for is always there. They are like fish swimming in the ocean, dying of thirst.

The water that could quench their thirst is everywhere. They only need to let it in, but they don't know how.

Many Have Closed Their Hearts

We connect to this larger field of love through our hearts. But sadly, many people have closed their hearts as a way to protect themselves from being hurt. While it certainly protects them from rejection, it numbs their hearts, disconnecting them from love. Cut off, they feel alone, alienated — and afraid.

Feeling alone and separate is the opposite of love. Karen Goldman, a contemporary American poet, writes:

> The feeling of separateness creates a volcano of pain in every human heart, liable to erupt. To ease the pressures of our lives we must open our hearts to each other and to ourselves, and know that within the love we will discover who and what we are and reclaim our connection to everyone.[3]

Feeling separate and unloved causes anger, depression and despair. When these emotions are suppressed, they are stored in the human body with grave consequences.

Many studies show that prolonged hostility:

* suppresses the immune system
* causes hypertension
* increases the risk of heart disease
* speeds aging

Love Heals

The antidote is love. It is profoundly healing emotionally and physically. While you probably know the healing power of love from your lifetime of experience, until recently very little research has measured the beneficial effects of positive emotions on health.

Dr. David McClelland, a Harvard psychologist and an influential scientist in the field of motivational psychology, was one of the first to study how care, compassion and altruism enhanced the immune system. When he had students watch a videotape of Mother Teresa working with the poor in Calcutta, he found it increased secretions of IgA, the antibody in saliva that protects against colds and upper respiratory infections. When the students viewed a film about Attila the Hun, the Mongol conqueror, their levels of IgA dropped.[4]

Recent studies have gone further to show the benefits of positive emotions. Researchers have found when individuals focused on emotions of caring and love, their hearts reflected an increased ordering in heart rhythm patterns which showed more harmony and efficiency in the cardiovascular system.

While this improved the functioning of the heart, it also influenced the whole body, since the heart produces a strong electromagnetic field of energy that surrounds the entire body, broadcasting its electrical information to every cell.[5]

Opening Your Heart

Thinking of someone easy to love is a way to open your heart. Choose a person or pet who you love unconditionally — without judgements. Bask in the glow of love you are giving and receiving.

Don't select a relationship that has ended, if recalling it makes you sad. While you'll remember the loving times, you may bump up against the sadness.

If the first person you pick doesn't elicit love, choose another, until you have someone you love and who loves you. Many people often recall the love of someone who has died. That is fine.

Don't confuse love with sexual desire. While you certainly can feel intense sensual passion for the one you love, this exercise is designed to open your heart by recalling love.

Angel or Spiritual Being

If you prefer, imagine a guardian angel or a spiritual figure who embodies qualities of divine love, such as Christ, Buddha or Mohammed.

Perhaps you'll want to commune with a feminine spiritual being. Think of the Mother Mary of the

Christian tradition, Shakti, the Hindu goddess, Kuan Yin, the beloved Chinese Goddess of Mercy, or the Green Tara, a Goddess of Tibetan Buddhism.

As the sun rises, the prayers and practice of the Green Tara are done on a daily basis in most Tibetan monasteries. She is the embodiment of the loving qualities of all the Buddhas, representing the compassion of the Cosmic Mother. As such, she has the power to heal and console.

If you choose a spiritual figure, feel his or her unconditional love streaming to you and feel your love or devotion flowing back.

When I was giving a lecture on self-healing for the Institute of Noetic Sciences in New York City, a woman in the back of the room raised her hand and said, "I am having heart surgery in a month and I have never felt loved. I've always loved people who didn't love me. What do I imagine since I don't have a memory to recall?"

Taken aback by her situation and candor, I answered, "You will have to imagine how it would feel to love someone who loves you. Just as your ideal place can be an actual place or one you create, the same is true in thinking of a person, a pet or a divine being who is easy to love. If the memory is not there, create it."

Imagine being loved. If you imagine it vividly enough, you will feel loved. You can create any feeling. The choice is always yours.

Oneness

Next I'll ask you to remember a time you felt a sense of oneness — a time you felt connected to something larger than yourself. Maybe you experienced it in nature, feeling the vibrancy of being one with everything — the earth, trees and sky. You may also have had a sense of oneness playing golf, jogging, listening to music or being with someone you love.

Sometimes this experience happens while looking at something you find beautiful, such as a flower or a sunrise. As you gaze at it — you merge, becoming one with it. In that moment, you have connected with the flow of life.

The Chinese call this seamless flow of life the Tao. In the sixth century B.C., the Chinese mystic Lao Tzu wrote about the Tao — the essence of life from which all forms spring into being.

If the experience of oneness is unfamiliar, continue imagining love flowing between you and another person or being. Whether you experience love or oneness, both create the biochemistry that speeds healing.

Healing Light

After you've bathed in the oneness or love, I'll ask you to imagine a vibrant, healing light flowing in through the top of your head, filling your body as it flows down to your toes.

Feel and see the light flowing through every cell in your body, placing every cell in harmony. Some people see a light. Some feel it and others experience a light intertwined with love. Let your experience be whatever it is. Don't try to change it. Let it evolve with daily practice.

Healing Process

Now that you are in a deep state of relaxation, you are ready to picture your healing. The CD guides you through visualizing three images related to your recuperation. The next chapter, Step 2: Visualize Your Healing, helps you develop your personal imagery.

The CD ends: "In a moment I am going to count from one to five. At the count of five, you can do what you would like to do next."

Often by the end of the relaxation, people feel so peaceful they just want to linger in the tranquility.

Linger as long as you like, knowing that it is healing, both emotionally and physically.

If your heart is filled with love, keep your attention on your heart. Experience the fullness and the flow of the love. The more you do this, the more you'll increase your capacity to love and be loved. In the process, you'll have discovered how you can call up the love that is always in your heart.

If you need to cook dinner or write a report, see if you can do it, remaining connected to the peace.

Insomnia

If you ever have insomnia, there is a completely different way to use the relaxation as a way to go to sleep. Stay awake as you listen to the CD. But when you come to the end of it, let yourself become very drowsy. Turn off the CD — drifting off to sleep, surrounded by love.

If you have trouble waking up in the night and can't fall back to sleep, use the CD in the same way. Keep the CD or iPod beside your bed.

Use Track 3 of the CD so it turns off as you fall asleep. If you use Track 1 and fall asleep, when Track 2 begins it would wake you up when you want to sleep.

If you sleep with someone, use headphones to avoid waking them. With practice, it will become easier to relax — falling back to sleep, embraced by love.

Summary

Step 1
Relax to Feel Peaceful

1. Knowing how to relax is one of the best ways to cope with the stress of surgery.

2. Of all medical problems, 85% are caused by stress. When you are anxious, you produce excess levels of stress hormones, such as cortisone and the catecholamines, which diminish the functioning of your immune system.

3. Your immune system is your body's natural defense system against illness. It is coordinated and controlled by T-cells that are produced in your thymus gland. While stress reduces T-cell counts, medical research shows that relaxation increases them, strengthening your immune system.

4. When you are afraid, your body shifts into a "fight-or-flight" response. This is a natural response, but living in a state of alarm for days or weeks before surgery will exhaust you and suppress your immune system and could lead to illness.

5. Learning how to relax gives you a way to stop the "fight-or-flight" response. Feeling calm also creates the complex biochemistry that relaxes your muscles,

enhances your immune system and helps you feel peaceful.

6. The first level of relaxation is letting go of physical tension, such as the tension of a clenched jaw, tight shoulder muscles or an overall sense of stress. The second level helps you let go of emotions that are stressful.

7. When you are more deeply relaxed, you may feel a sense of connectedness or oneness. People often experience this in nature, feeling one with the whole landscape — the earth, the trees and the sky. You may have felt connected to something larger than yourself while listening to music, meditating or being with someone you love.

Tennis players call it being "in the zone." Joggers know it when they feel "lighter than air, able to run forever — almost like flying."

8. Philosophers call this sense of connectedness or oneness the "transcendental dimension" because you have transcended your everyday state of being. Psychologists call it the "transpersonal dimension," meaning beyond the personal.

9. As you listen to the Relaxation CD, stress can be released physically or emotionally. You may also experience a wave of emotion as it arises and releases. Welcome it instead of resisting it.

10. The more often you use the Relaxation CD each day, the sooner your stress-related symptoms will diminish or disappear. These may include tension headaches, migraines and anxiety.

11. All it takes is practice. Choose one or two times of the day to use the CD. Schedule the times in your calendar.

12. Create a support system for developing this skill. Ask a friend or family member to learn the art of relaxation with you. Or at the very least, ask a friend if you can check in each day to say you have used the CD.

13. Use headphones to give you your own private healing atmosphere at home and in the hospital.

14. If you get sleepy listening to the CD, bring your mind back to consciousness so you can follow the directed relaxation.

15. Imagine yourself in your ideal place rather than looking at a picture of yourself there. If your ideal place is a favorite beach — feel the warmth of the sun, smell the sea air and hear the waves breaking on the sand now.

16. Think of a person or pet who is easy to love. Let your mind go back to a specific time you felt a great deal of love, feeling your love flow to the person or

pet and feel his or her love flow back to you. Experience all the emotions as if they were happening now.

17. Remember a time you felt a sense of oneness. If the experience of oneness is unfamiliar, continue imagining the love flowing between you and the other person or pet.

18. Imagine a vibrant, healing light flowing in through the top of your head, filling your body as it flows all the way down to your toes.

19. At the end of the CD, linger as long as you like in the tranquility, knowing that it is healing both physically and emotionally. If you want to cook dinner or write a report, do it remaining connected to the peace or love in your heart.

20. If you have insomnia, there is a different way to use the relaxation process to go to sleep. Stay awake as you listen to the CD. But when you come to the end, let yourself become drowsy. Turn off the recorder — falling asleep surrounded by love.

21. If you wake up in the middle of the night and have trouble going back to sleep, use the CD in the same way — falling asleep embraced by love.

22. Add your ideas:

Step 2

Visualize Your Healing

For visualization *is* the way we think.
Before words, images were.

— Don Gerrard

You can help your recovery by visualizing your ideal surgical outcome. Let the imagery fill your mind, heart and being.

Use your senses to make it come alive, the way you imagined your ideal place of relaxation. <u>Feel</u> the warmth of the sun, <u>smell</u> the fresh sea air and <u>hear</u> the waves breaking on the sand. You'll notice how different this is from imagining a two-dimensional picture in your mind.

At Harvard University, research by psychologist,

Dr. Mary Jasnoski has shown that while relaxation enhanced immune defenses against upper respiratory infections, adding visualization increased people's immunity.[1]

Don't use your mental force to push away a negative image with a positive one. This is like putting beautiful wallpaper on top of a stain. Eventually the old stain bleeds through.

At first, it's all right if a part of you doesn't quite believe your positive visualization. With daily practice, you'll discover that soon you will believe it. At that point, you'll experience an ease with which you see and feel the healed outcome.

Allow Healing

It's a peaceful sense of surrender that allows healing rather than commanding it. Surrendering does not mean giving up. Instead it's a letting go — an entrusting.

Focus on the healed outcome of your operation rather than on the surgical process of getting there. Ask your doctor to describe, and even draw a picture of the desired surgical result. If any of your surgeon's words evoke negative images, ask him or her, to use other words that are more positive.

Nancy Claflin of Belmont, Massachusetts, wanted to do everything she could to minimize her pain and help her healing, following shoulder surgery. She was very worried. Several friends, and even her own surgeon, had warned her that she would feel a great deal of pain after her operation. To reduce the pain, she asked her anesthesiologist to say the therapeutic statements during surgery.

To further promote her recovery, Nancy called me to work out the precise healing images she wanted to visualize before and after surgery. She recounted that a good friend, a renowned hip surgeon, had explained that her shoulder's torn rotator cuff probably looked like frayed ropes. He described how her surgeon would be reattaching these frayed ropes, her tendons, to her shoulder bone.

Nancy didn't like the image of "frayed ropes." She said, "I've been around enough boats to know it's impossible to pull old ropes together into a strong one."

To get a more positive image, she called her surgeon's resident and asked him to describe her operation. Nancy said, "Instead of frayed ropes, he talked about securing my strong, pink biceps tendons to my shoulder bone."

His description gave her vivid, positive images. Nancy used them in two ways. When she noticed worries about her operation popping into her mind, she replaced the worries with pictures of her healed shoulder. In addition, twice a day, she used the Relaxation CD to calm and guide her through visualizing her surgical outcome.

Focus on the Healed Outcome

In anticipating surgery, Nancy didn't dwell on the surgical process of cutting and drilling. Instead she imagined her end result: "pink, strong tendons securely attached to her shoulder bone."

Create a beautiful image of the healed outcome that makes you feel peaceful whenever you call up the image. Don't create a bloody horror movie of the medical details.

When worries about your operation pop into your mind, switch the worries to pictures of your healed outcome, much like changing the channel on television. You can change your thoughts in an instant.

As you pay attention to your thoughts, you'll notice how often you create pictures of worry and fear. If you let your mind run on like this, you'll find these worries lead to more and more worries.

When you worry, you create images of the very thing you don't want to happen. If you worry long enough, you generate an ongoing movie of fear, which runs on its own in your subconscious, giving you a pervasive sense of fear and dread. Watch your thoughts.

It takes as much effort to have negative thoughts as it does to have healing ones. Do you want to scare yourself with your fears or comfort yourself with healing thoughts?

You can't control everything in your life, but one thing you have a great deal of control over is your own mind. You are the producer and editor of your thoughts and emotions; and you are your own audience.

Seeing a positive outcome doesn't mean denying your negative thoughts and feelings. You acknowledge they are there, but you choose to dwell on the positive ones. It means genuinely becoming optimistic by deliberately rehearsing the positive imagery until it is yours.

At a certain point, you'll discover that you believe it. You'll feel a kind of surrender when it no longer is an effort to imagine your successful surgical outcome.

Comforting Feeling

Following surgery as Nancy had hoped, she felt only mild discomfort. When several nurses told her that she was using much less pain medication than other patients having the same operation, Nancy explained that she believed she had lessened the pain by asking her anesthesiologist to say the therapeutic statements during surgery.

Undoubtedly, Nancy's belief in the statements, coupled with her anticipation of less pain, and the statements themselves, all contributed to diminishing her pain.

Excited by this tangible result, Nancy telephoned me from her room at Massachusetts General Hospital to discuss what else she could do to influence her recovery. In response, I offered to lead her through a guided imagery exercise.

Guided Imagery Exercise

The exercise would let her shoulder symbolically "talk" to her, explaining what feelings would comfort it and enhance its healing. Although her shoulder couldn't literally talk, the exercise would give it a voice so that Nancy could dialogue with it.

To center and calm Nancy, I led her through the relaxation exercise. Since she had used the CD at home, several times a day for two weeks before her operation, Nancy was skilled at going into deep states of relaxation. When she was deeply relaxed, I said, "Let an image of your shoulder appear."

Nancy said, "I have an image of it."

I said, "Good. Ask it: What comforting feeling do you want me to give you?" Nancy answered, "It wants a feeling of softness and protection."

I responded, "Ask: How many times a day do you want me to give you this feeling?"

Nancy said, "It wants it for 10 seconds, whenever I think about my shoulder, and three times a day for five minutes when I am very relaxed."

As we continued talking, Nancy broke in, "I just did it. I gave it that feeling. I'm being softer and more protective of my shoulder whenever I shift my position."

For two weeks, whenever she thought about her shoulder, Nancy gave it feelings of "softness and protection" for 10 seconds. In addition, three times a day she scheduled the five-minute healing sessions.

Settled in a comfortable chair, she listened to the CD, taking about 15 minutes to reach a deep state of relaxation. As the CD continued, it guided her through five minutes of visualizing "pink, strong tendons securely attached to her shoulder bone." She also felt the "softness and protection" soothing her shoulder. Playfully, she imagined oiling the joint with the lubricant WD-40®.

Other times in the day when she worried about her shoulder, she switched her worries to images of healing for one minute. By repeating the imagery, she created a pervasive healing theme that reverberated throughout her consciousness.

Even her dreams became ones of healing. When she recalled a dream, often it was about her shoulder's ongoing recuperation.

Nancy's surgeon had told her to plan on four weeks of recovery. That meant four weeks of having her arm immobilized in a sling. Just before her two-week checkup, Nancy called me, saying, "My shoulder feels so good, as if it's healed."

The next day when Nancy's doctor tested her shoulder's range of motion, he found it had healed two weeks ahead of schedule. The X-rays also showed that Nancy had experienced a degree of healing normally expected to take four weeks.

Thrilled with her doctor's news, Nancy was eager to begin physical therapy to strengthen her atrophied muscles and regain the use of her shoulder. With her physical therapist, Nancy set new goals to visualize.

Now that the muscles and tendons of her shoulder were getting stronger from lifting weights, she pictured herself easily picking up her dog, a collie named Missy. Before surgery and physical therapy, lifting her dog, or even her binoculars when she was bird-watching, would have been impossible.

Athletes Use Visualization

Physical therapists and athletes know the benefits of using visualization techniques to increase the effectiveness of physical training and conditioning. Amateur and professional athletes use mental training to envision hitting a home run, shooting a basket or doing a perfect high dive. Probably every Olympic medalist has hundreds of times visualized winning a gold medal.

During physical therapy, when people think of themselves as physically limited, due to an injury or surgery, therapists often urge patients to change their self-image, imagining themselves recovered and vital again. Doing so speeds up people's recoveries because they are more optimistic, more determined and less willing to give up during their physical workouts.

Interestingly, when the British runner Roger Bannister made history by becoming the first person to run a mile in less than four minutes in 1954, he accomplished a feat that had been thought to be physiologically impossible. But once this psychological barrier had been broken, within 12 months 52 other runners ran the mile in less than four minutes.

Clearly, the only limitation had been in the runners' own minds, believing it was impossible.

Find your own psychological barriers. What do you believe you can't do or be? Imagining yourself without that specific limitation is often the first step to moving beyond it. Once you have mentally gone beyond it, a door may open or you will be receptive to information that could move you further along.

Feeling Is an Aspect of Visualization

When you envision your healing process, feel as well as see the comforting feeling flow through the recovering part of your body.

Involving your kinesthetic sense strengthens your imagery. Nancy saw and felt the "softness and protection" permeating her shoulder. Similarly, when athletes mentally rehearse, they feel each step of their tennis serve or golf swing.

When Norman Cousins, author of *Anatomy of an Illness*, the story of his remarkable recovery from a crippling disease, broke his arm, he envisioned and felt the warmth of the increased flow of blood bringing nutrients to his knitting bone.

After using the imagery in a relaxed state of mind for a number of weeks, several times a day, he urged his doctor to X-ray his arm. The X-rays showed that his bone had healed several weeks sooner than expected.

Talking to Your Body

Before and after your operation, ask the part of your body that is healing what comforting feeling it wants you to give it.

* **Find a private place that's peaceful.**
* **Become calm, using the Relaxation CD, meditation or self-hypnosis.**
* **Imagine the part of your body you want to heal.**

Some people conjure up a realistic picture from a medical textbook; others prefer to let a symbolic image appear. Some even have characterizations. One woman imagined her liver sitting in a rocking chair, telling her it felt irritated. It wanted to be lulled and rocked until it felt calm.

While most people find it easy to use imagery, some ask, "If I'm not good at visualizing, how can I make this process work?" Draw a picture or a cartoon of the healing process that you imagine is taking place. Ask your doctor to draw a picture. Either one will give you an image to conjure up.

Actually, you don't have to visualize your elbow to have it "talk" to you. Just ask it the questions and the answers will come. We all have an inner wisdom, an inner knowing or Higher Self called "intuition." It is this faculty you are using to "talk" to your body.

When you are relaxed, your rational mind is put at rest, letting your intuition answer the questions. Remember when your rational mind made a list of all the reasons to make a decision, but your intuition said to make a different decision? It is this intuitive voice you are using.

Be still and open to the answer. You may hear a voice that is similar to your own imagination talking. When you are really in touch with your inner knowing, this voice will be clear and direct. Instead of hearing a voice, you may have a sense of certainty, the experience of "knowing you know." **It may be a gut feeling or a knowing in your heart.**

Each time this happens, you will learn more about how your inner wisdom talks to you. The more that you listen to your intuition and act on it, the more practiced you will be at identifying it.

It is different from the other inner voices of doubt, worry or self-criticism that you may hear. Your inner knowing never puts you down or ridicules you. Instead it is compassionate and clear.

Trust Your Intuition

Rational Western society gives women more permission to listen to their intuition. However, a survey of men, who were CEOs of several American companies, revealed how much men rely on their intuition when making business decisions. When asked, "How do you make important decisions?" The executives responded in a similar way. They said that if their gut feelings was "Yes" and their minds came to the same conclusion, it was an easy decision.

But when faced with the conflict of their guts saying "Yes" and their minds saying "No," they always followed their guts. They also reported often using facts to validate their intuitions. In board meetings, they were reluctant to admit that their decisions were based on gut feelings.[2]

Your illness or physical condition is already trying to "talk" to you, telling you that something is amiss. Your intuition knows what is out of balance and causing a health problem. Allow yourself to hear what it is. Ask questions and listen for the answers.

Look for Emotional Component
While surgery will correct the physical problem, you'll want to look for the underlining emotional component that may be causing it. Often there is one.

By "talking" to your body before surgery and releasing any emotions that may be involved, your healing process will be much easier after surgery.

And there is always the possibility that your condition may improve or heal completely without surgery.

Unresolved Grief and Rage

When Ginger Marley of Hartford, Connecticut, needed surgery to remove an ovarian cyst, she called me to make an appointment to release her unresolved grief and rage from an abortion two years earlier.

Although the abortion had been medically necessary, she had felt rushed into it by her doctor. She had not had enough time to do the inner work of emotionally releasing the fetus before it was physically removed.

Her current surgeon now was encouraging her to release the trauma of the abortion before undergoing surgery to remove the ovarian cyst. Otherwise the emotional distress of the abortion could be retriggered, complicating her recovery from the upcoming operation.

During our individual session, Ginger grieved the loss of her unborn child — sobbing uncontrollably until the sobs were gone. Next came her anger, expressed in screams of outrage.

Once the rage had been released, Ginger was calm. I sensed that unconsciously she withheld energy from her pelvis. To understand the cause, I suggested she ask her uterus, "How do I feel about you?"

It answered, "You believe I betrayed you when you could not get pregnant after the abortion."

Ginger said, "That's right. I began to hate my uterus when it became difficult to get pregnant."

As Ginger talked to it, her uterus asked her to fill it with love and imagine the cyst getting smaller. As her love flowed into her uterus, she realized it was her ally. It had already given her two wonderful children. After using the relaxation process with her healing imagery, twice a day, every day during the week before surgery, Ginger felt prepared for the operation to remove the cyst.

She recovered so quickly that she left the hospital two days earlier than planned — to the surprise of her health insurance provider, The Travelers.

Release the Part of Your Body with Love
If a part of your body will be removed, before surgery find your way to thank it and say good-bye. For example, Dr. Christiane Northrup tells patients, "Release the part with love and gratitude for what it has given you."

Dr. Northrup, a leading women's health advocate in America and Europe, is the author of *Women's Bodies, Women's Wisdom: Creating Physical and Emotional Health and Healing*. A ground-breaking medical guide, it empowers women to take control of their own physical, emotional and spiritual health.

Dr. Northrup writes, "A woman's health is directly tied up in the culture where she lives, her position in it and how she lives her life. The physical symptoms of reproductive or gynecological disorders communicate wisdom about women's lives, the issues they need to face and the changes they must make in order to heal and live fully."

"When women realize they are in a bad relationship or a dead-end career and work to change their attitudes and lives, concurrent changes will occur. Their infertility may be cured, cancer goes into remission and fibroids disappear."

Another example of emotionally preparing for surgery is offered by Dr. Mitchell Levine, an obstetrician and gynecologist in Arlington, Massachusetts. When patients need surgery, he asks them to go through a conscious process or ceremony at home to make peace with the procedure. If a fibroid is being removed, he asks the patient to imagine all traumatic memories from her life are being removed at the same time.

Dr. Levine finds that patients recover much faster when they have emotionally prepared for surgery.

Questions to Ask

As you begin a conversation with your body, your inner self's answers will lead you to ask the next obvious question and may even initiate a dialogue. You'll hear or intuitively know the answers. It's helpful to record them in a notebook.

Write down each answer before you go on to the next question. This level of truth will be more powerful if it is grounded in the written word and ultimately in your understanding and actions.

Once relaxed, let an image of the part that needs healing appear in your imagination. Usually this is easier if your eyes are closed. Experiment to see which way you prefer. Address each of the following questions to the image:

* **"What are you feeling?"**
* **"What is causing you to feel that way?"**
* **"What comforting feeling do you want me to give you?"**
* **"What color is the feeling?"**
* **"How many times a day and for how long do you want this feeling?"**
* **"Is there anything else you want to tell me?"**

Healing Imagery

A man scheduled for back surgery asked his lower back, "What emotion would comfort you?" It answered, "Emotional support." Recalling a time he felt believed in and supported, he bathed his back in this sensation before and after surgery.

Before surgery to remove fibroids, a woman asked her uterus, "What emotion would comfort you?" It said, "Love." Resting her hands on her pelvis, she felt warmth and love flowing from her hands into her uterus. After surgery, she soothed her uterus in the same way — with love.

Lesson in the Illness

Often there is a lesson in the illness. For example, a woman had a series of medical tests to find the cause of fatigue. When all the tests showed that her physical health was fine, she finally asked her inner self, "Why am I feeling so tired?"

The answer came back, "You, like everyone, connect to the world through your heart. Through it flows a great deal of energy. But when your heart is closed, your energy stops flowing. You need to love more — then you'll have plenty of energy."

Following her heart's request, she thought of each person she loved, letting her love flow to them, one at a time. At first there was only a trickle of emotion. As she envisioned the third person, the trickle became a stream of love.

She experienced a welling up of emotion. Its warmth spread across her chest. The more she actively sent out her love to each grandchild and friend, the more the flow increased.

While this filled her with love, she also discovered she had more physical energy. To keep her heart open, she developed a daily routine. Each morning when she woke up, while lying in bed, she took ten minutes to send love to the people she cared about most. Her practice primed the pump, getting love flowing again.

Throughout the day, she periodically focused her awareness on her heart, checking if it was closed, as had been her life-long habit. If it was, she took a few minutes to recall her grandchild. Imagining the child's smile always opened her heart.

Questions to Find the Lesson

If there might be a lesson in your illness, ask the involved part of your body, such as your lung, elbow or knee the following questions:

* **"Why are you sick?"**
* **"What are you are trying to tell me?"**
* **"What's out of balance in my life?"**
* **"What is causing the problem?"**

Next ask the part of your body, "What comforting emotion do you want me to give you?" If your hip wants to be given love or peace, put your hand on it, feeling the love or peace flowing from your hand into your hip.

If your hand cannot reach the part of your body that wants healing, place your attention on that area . With your thoughts, mentally send love or peace to it.

Depending on how often your body tells you it wants the comforting emotion, at a minimum give it that emotion for a few minutes two to three times a day or more if it would like it.

Use Relaxation CD Twice A Day

I recommend listening to the Relaxation CD twice a day for one to two weeks before surgery. Every time you use it, you'll shift yourself out of fear into feeling relaxed or if you're already calm into a deeper state of relaxation.

I'm often asked, "My surgery is a two months away, how soon should I start using the CD twice a day?" My answer is, "If you're feeling anxious about surgery, begin now. The sooner you start using it, the sooner you'll feel calmer and look forward to your surgery.

Even if you only have one day before your operation, using the CD will still help to reduce your anxiety before surgery. After surgery it will lessen your use of pain medication, help you sleep and speed your healing.

The CD guides you through progressive states of relaxation and gives you time to imagine three end-results. On the CD I suggest some healing imagery. But it is better if you visualize your personalized scene, feeling like the scene is happening now.

Your First End-Result

Your first end-result is about telling a friend or family members how comfortable you are feeling after you have left the recovery room. If it is day surgery, this scene will be at home.

If you'll be spending the night in the hospital, imagine what you'd like to say when you are settled in your hospital room.

Feel the soft pillows behind your shoulders. See your friend, spouse or children coming into your hospital room.

Feel their love for you and your love for them. Hear them asking, "How are you feeling?" Hear yourself saying, "I feel comfortable."

Don't say, "Thank God it is over." That is negative. Don't say, "I have no pain." Don't even use the word, "pain."

If they would hold your hand or gently stoke your forehead, feel that happening now. See a favorite family photograph on your bedside table. If you'd be comforted by flowers, see your favorite flowers.

Intensive Care Unit (ICU)

If you are having a surgery that requires your going to the Intensive Care Unit (ICU) instead of your hospital room, the scene of your first end-result will be in the ICU.

Ask if you'll be able to talk when your family visits you in the ICU. If you'll be intubated, having a tube in your throat that helps you breath but prevents you from talking, you won't be able to say, "I feel comfortable." But you can tell your family that you'll give them a thumbs up signal that means you feel comfortable and are doing well.

Day Surgery

If you're having day surgery and going home after leaving the recovery room, visualize your first end result at home. Feel surrounded by the love of your family and your love for them.

See the details of the room you'll be in. Hear your favorite music playing in the background. Smell something delicious cooking in the kitchen. Hear a family member asking, "How do you feel?" Visualize saying, "I feel comfortable."

Changing Your First End Result

After your first end-result happens, replace it with your next short term goal for healing. Ask your nurse "What's my goal for tomorrow?" He or she might say, "Walking to the end of the hallway and back."

Imagine you've done that and feel triumphant as you visualize your new first end-result.

Second End-Result
Your second end-result is a scene that means you are recovering well. You are not fully recovered but you know you are healing well. For example, you might say to a friend or your spouse, "I am feeling so well lets go out for dinner and a movie."

If you've had a hip-joint replacement, you might visualize taking a short walk with your spouse or good friend. Include all the details of what you see, hear, smell and feel. Imagine saying, "My hip feels strong." Feel like you are taking the walk now.

If you love to cook, you might want to imagine being in the kitchen cooking your favorite dish, smelling the aromas and feeling the strength in the part of your body that is healing. Have someone you love in the scene. It might be a spouse, friend, grandchild or beloved dog. Feel your love for them and their love for you.

Your Third End-Result
Your third end-result is a scene in which you are completely healed doing something you love.

Make this a scene that holds your passion. That passion is the key to what you visualize. Life is precious. You don't want to live it doing something you are lukewarm about.

Create the scene in the present. Feel it happening now. Imagine you are recovered. This is quite different from longing to be recovered.

If your passion is tennis, imagine vigorously playing a game. Hear the bong of the ball as you hit it. Smell your sunburn lotion. See the blue sky and the pine trees lining the court. Feel exhilarated and experience strength in the part of your body that is healed, your shoulder, hip, spine, knee or wrist.

Being in the scene makes your imagery more alive. This is different from seeing a picture of yourself playing tennis.

Healing Imagery for Cancer
If you are having surgery to remove cancer, put your third end-result far in the future. If you are 45, have your third end-result be a scene when you are 65 or 75 years old. If you are 45 now, would you worry if you knew you were going to be 80 years old?

I remember doing a one-hour workshop with a woman in her 40s who was facing a mastectomy. For her third end-result, she visualized her 80th birthday party. In her scene she had just come from working out at the gym and loved how strong and healthy she felt. She saw and heard her friends and family singing, "Happy Birthday to You" as she blew out the candles on her cake. She saw a big 80 written in blue frosting on the cake.

When she felt afraid, she visualized her 80th birthday for one minute. It calmed her and gave her a way to shift herself out of fear and into the positive feelings.

Visualize for One Minute

If you listen to the Relaxation CD for 20 minutes twice a day but worry the rest of the day, your worry will cancel out your positive imagery.

To prevent this from happening, realize you create all your thoughts. Every time you start to worry about the surgery, take one minute to enjoy your third end-result, feeling like it is happening now.

For the first day or two, you will need to be very persistent to turn away from the worry and instead focus on feeling your third end-result. The more you do it the easier it becomes.

Use CD after Surgery and before PT

After surgery, listen to the CD several times a day. If you're having physical therapy (PT), listening to the CD 30 minutes before it will relax your muscles, allowing for more range of motion.

Many orthopedic surgeons have been pleased and surprised by the excellent range of motion patients had in a shoulder, knee or hip joint when they used this book and CD before and after surgery.

Visualize throughout the Day

 * If you go to work by train or bus, use 20 minutes of the commute to listen to the CD and imagine your end-results.

 * As you wait for an elevator or a red traffic light or while you wash the dishes, take a few moments to visualize yourself fully recovered.

 * Put a small, colored dot on your watch. Whenever you look at it, the dot reminds you to visualize your healing for one minute. Most of us look at our watches 20 to 30 times a day. As a result, your day becomes filled with 20 to 30 minutes of healing images that speed recovery.

 * In addition to imagining end-results during the day, some people also like to envision them when they wake up in the morning, others as they drop off to sleep.

 * As you go to sleep, tell your body, "All night, while I am sleeping, healing is taking place." See and feel the healing as you fall asleep. You will sleep more deeply all night because you are relaxed.

Believe in Your Medicine

If your doctor has prescribed medication, do you imagine the healing qualities of your pills or wince as you swallow them, afraid of negative side effects? **What you believe about your medicine powerfully alters its effectiveness.**

For example, the loss of hair sometimes associated with chemotherapy was experienced by 30 percent of the people in a control group, who never even received chemotherapy. Instead they were given only a placebo, an inactive substance used in experiments to compare it with the chemically active drug being tested.

Clearly, it was the power of the beliefs, as well as the expectation of the negative side effects of chemotherapy, that caused the loss of hair. *The World Journal of Surgery* published these findings, reporting on a study of the effectiveness of different types of chemotherapy.

If you are ambivalent about your medication, find a way to let go of your doubts and wholeheartedly embrace its healing properties. Studies have shown that people who are optimistic about their medical treatments usually recover sooner.

However, this does not mean that you should override an intuitive feeling that your medication is harmful. If you have such a nagging feeling, discuss your concerns with your doctor. It is possible that your intuition is correct.

How Long Will It Take to Heal?

Your healing process is influenced by many things, including your state of health, the quality of treatment and your beliefs. If you believe that the more serious an operation is the longer it takes to heal, then your recuperation may take longer. But if you can find a way to change your beliefs, thinking you will get well sooner, your positive expectation will help you heal sooner.

Your doctor's idea of "normal" healing time is based on allowing the body's natural healing process to take its course. However, if you are relaxed and visualizing your healing process, you are creating the biochemistry that speeds healing.

By comparison, if you are anxious and afraid, you create the biochemistry that suppresses your immune system, very possibly lengthening your recuperation.

Usually your doctor will tell you a range of time or the maximum amount of time that it will take to recover based on other people's experiences. Each person's rate of recovery is different. Ask what is a possible shorter time, and use that information to change your beliefs in a way that is reasonable.

People with Good Recoveries

Ask your doctor for the names of two or three people, who have recovered well from the operation you will be having. Your surgeon's secretary usually can get the patients' permission for you to contact them. You'll be inspired by their stories.

Dr. Joseph Moskal, a surgeon at the Roanoke Orthopedic Center in Virginia, asks his patients who are excellent examples of recovery from hip-replacement surgery to meet with his new patients before their operations. The recovered patients offer real-life encouragement to the people facing surgery.

Do You Deserve to Recover Successfully?

Carole Angermeir felt a pang of guilt when I asked her to imagine seeing clearly after eye surgery to remove a cataract. When I said, "Why do you feel guilty?" She immediately answered, "My mother and two aunts are legally blind. If I can see again out of my cloudy eye, I'll be disloyal because I'll be leaving them behind."

As an anthropologist with a pilot's license, Carole had been instrumental in bringing eyesight to thousands of people. She had helped to fund and establish eye clinics in 18 developing countries, including several floating clinics in the Amazon and several mobile units in the bush country of Kenya.

Now as she faced eye surgery, she acknowledged her life-long conflict of being different from her mother.

Safe to See
As she turned this issue over in her mind and soul, she realized she didn't need blurry vision to be a part of her family. It was safe for her eyesight to be restored.

This realization freed her to imagine a successful outcome for her operation. During the week before surgery, several times a day, she imagined her end-result: seeing clearly again and feeling happy about it.

On the morning of her day-surgery, Carole used self-hypnosis to calm herself in the waiting room at New York Hospital-Cornell Medical Center in New York City. Leaning her head against the wall and stretching out her legs, she guided herself into a state of deep relaxation. Imagining herself on a favorite beach in Quintana Roo, Mexico, she felt the warmth of the sun. She was so calm, she felt as if she were floating.

Carole had asked three friends to send her tranquility for the half-hour before surgery. At the appointed time, she smiled as a whoosh of tranquility surrounded her.

Carole said, "By the time I went into the operating room, I was blissful."

Throughout the operation, during which she was awake, her years of training in self-hypnosis helped her stay calm. Having assisted at hundreds of cataract operations, in makeshift tents in developing countries, she knew every step of the procedure.

Soothed by Swirling Pink and Blue Clouds

During her recovery at home, whenever her eye ached in the middle of the night, she soothed it with images of swirling pink and blue clouds and fell back to sleep. Each day she took several times to envision the healing.

Although her eye was healing ahead of schedule, it still did not have the full improvement she had imagined as her successful recovery. She didn't settle for the mediocre result. Instead she persisted in asking her doctor questions, such as, "What could be causing the blur in my vision?"

When her surgeon gave her answers that didn't satisfy her, Carole talked to his surgical resident. He explained that two temporary sutures might be holding her new lens too tightly in place, causing the blur.

Carole suggested that removing the sutures might restore her vision. With her urging, the resident took out the first suture. But her vision was still blurred. Again, she encouraged him to remove the second suture. Within an hour of snipping it free, she could see.

Carole is an example of a person who listened to her intuitive knowing and had the courage to follow it. Urging her doctor to proceed further resulted in her restored vision.

Preparing for Brain Surgery

Marshall Gould was facing surgery to remove a tumor on his pituitary gland. He was terrified of the impending 15-hour brain operation at Mount Sinai Hospital in New York City. The tumor was pressing on nerves leading to his vocal cords, making it hard to speak. His voice had been squeezed to a whisper. He could swallow only liquefied food.

As we talked on the phone about how he could relax, I discovered that 25 years ago he had learned self-hypnosis as a way to stop smoking. At my suggestion, he used hypnosis to shift himself out of the fight-or-flight response.

Once relaxed, he imagined playing a round of golf. He loved the beauty and peace of a golf course. It was his ideal place of relaxation.

His operation was scheduled in two days. For 10 minutes of every hour that he was awake, I asked him to stretch out in his hospital bed, using self-hypnosis to relax his whole body and imagine a game of golf.

When I talked to him the next day, he sounded like a different person. His voice had lost its raspiness. He felt peaceful and could cope better with the thought of the operation. He could swallow easily. In fact, he had just enjoyed eating his first full meal in a week.

Bliss

He told me, "When my thoughts stop, I feel a kind of bliss. It's almost like Nirvana. It feels so good that I let the 10 minutes become 20, as I float in bliss. What is it?" I explained that when he quiets his mind, there is a spacious peace and a vast void. It is pure awareness.

Now that he could calm himself, I asked him to imagine the tumor getting smaller and smaller and disappearing. At first he laughed at my suggestion, saying, "You have got to be kidding. You mean my thoughts could influence this thing and make it smaller?"

Although he was very skeptical, he figured it would not hurt to try. As he walked the halls of Mount Sinai Hospital, he pictured a white light flowing into the tumor, disintegrating it. He talked to the tumor, saying, "Your days are numbered. It's time for you to leave."

He Went into Surgery Relaxed

The morning of surgery, Marshall felt more relaxed and optimistic. His wife was greatly relieved seeing the change in him. To deal with her fears about the long operation, she put her feet up on a chair and listened to the Relaxation CD. It washed away the strain of the hours of waiting for the operation to be completed.

The operation was successful. The tumor was benign. During his recuperation in the hospital and at home, whenever he was agitated, Marshall listened to the Relaxation CD to calm himself and visualize his healing.

Whenever he worried about his recovery, he imagined light flowing through his body, aiding his healing. At night as he fell asleep, he pictured the healing continuing through the night. Using the mind-body techniques, Marshall participated in his several months of recovery, regaining health well ahead of schedule.

Mind-Body Techniques

While most people use the techniques of relaxation and visualization to prepare for surgery and facilitate their recovery, some have utilized these methods to heal — avoiding surgery.

The self-healing tools in this book are meant to be used in conjunction with your doctor and conventional medicine. Ask your surgeon if you might have a medical condition that would improve by putting them into practice.

If your operation is several weeks or even a month away, you have nothing to lose and everything to gain by learning to relax and envision your healing as you prepare for surgery.

Don't fall into the trap of creating the duality of alternative versus conventional medicine — debating which to use. Instead, use the best of both worlds.

Your Thoughts Are Powerful Medicine

Your focused thoughts, images and emotions are powerful medicine. Utilizing them, you are helping to push the envelope of a frontier, the field of mind-body medicine. The medical evidence of your results will inspire others to do the same. I invite you to send me an email at peggy@HealFaster.com about your experiences.

To encourage you, here are examples of two people who avoided surgery by listening to their inner knowing and harnessing their innate powers of self-healing.

Illness can be a great impetus. When we are sick, we may finally be willing to consult our inner wisdom, which has the power to bring our lives back to harmony and health.

New Bone Growth

Patricia Morris, a computer programmer in Short Hills, New Jersey, had broken her finger. Twelve weeks after the injury, X-rays showed that no healing was taking place. To encourage bone growth, her surgeon had recommended inserting a steel pin to join the two fractured pieces of bone.

Although Patricia had called me to help her prepare for surgery scheduled in three weeks, I suggested that she might get the bone growing again by visualizing the healing process. If she could stimulate bone growth, she could avoid surgery.

Patricia had broken the ring finger on her right hand. She had worn an engagement ring on this finger until her fiancé had suddenly broken their engagement. The next week Patricia had an accident, breaking her finger.

I explained that if she relaxed into an altered state of consciousness, her healing imagery would have more of an impact than it would in her waking state. As I guided her through the relaxation process, she said, "I feel as if I'm floating."

To find out why the normal healing had not taken place for 12 weeks, I showed Patricia how to dialogue with her finger, giving her specific questions to ask.

The first was, "What are you feeling?" It responded, "Alone and cut off." When she asked, "Why?" It said, "You have isolated me, treating me like something outside of yourself."

Patricia said, "That is right. My way of dealing with my finger and the broken engagement was to block them out, never thinking about them." She went on to say, "I wasn't going to let it get me down."

As she talked she started to cry, feeling an ache in her heart. Patricia realized that blocking out her thoughts and numbing her emotions had been her way to avoid the heartache of the broken engagement.

Next I asked her, "What feeling does your finger want you to give it?" She answered, "Love" — as a beam of it arced from her heart down her arm to her injured finger.

An important part of Patricia's healing was allowing her heart to open and love again. She had closed it to avoid her sadness. Now her first attempts at love were to let it permeate her own finger.

Whenever worries about her finger popped into her mind, I asked her to envision the bone knitting for one minute. This would change her mental habit of disassociating from her broken finger.

In addition, I asked her twice a day for 20 minutes to use the CD to guide her into a deep state of relaxation in which she visualized her bone healing.

After 10 days of visualization, her doctor's X-ray showed new bone growth. Encouraged by this result, her surgeon suggested delaying the operation for two more weeks, hoping the healing would persist.

Two weeks later when her doctor X-rayed her finger, he saw more healing, which he found "highly unusual." As a result, he recommended canceling surgery. In another month, her finger had healed.

Why the Mind-Body Techniques Worked

It's understandable that Patricia's bone would heal once she stopped disassociating from her finger. Her healing process was the exact opposite of what she had been doing.

Instead of ignoring her finger, she learned to give it attention, visualizing the bones knitting together and soothing them with love.

It is doubtful that Patricia's bone would have healed so fast, or at all, if she had only used the healing imagery twice a day and the rest of the day resorted to her defense of blocking out all thoughts of her physical and emotional injury.

The key to her recovery was sending healing to her finger whenever the thought of it came into her mind. It was a simple but profound act. It reestablished the natural flow of energy to her arm and finger. With time, this allowed her broken finger to mend as well as her broken heart.

Recovery from Gallbladder Attacks

Indiana Nelson, a writer and painter in Tucson, Arizona, called me when her doctor suggested she might need to have her gallbladder removed. For months she had been having painful gallbladder attacks once every two weeks.

During a phone session I guided her through a process of relaxation, showing her how her gallbladder could "talk" to her.

She asked her gallbladder what it was feeling. It explained that she was grieving. Her two sons, ages 17 and 19, were about to leave home to go away to school. She knew that her two boys had to leave her, but she still felt betrayed. She had stored those feelings of betrayal in her gallbladder.

When she asked her gallbladder what comforting feeling it wanted, it said, "Waves of gentle love and a little bit of chocolate once a day."

It explained that food represented love. The bland gallbladder diet that she followed made her feel deprived at just the time the love of her sons was leaving. Her gallbladder said that to heal the betrayal, she needed to feel loved and to love what she was eating.

For three weeks, she gave her gallbladder "waves of gentle love" for 10 minutes, four times a day. Once a day she slowly ate one Hershey's chocolate kiss. And at each meal of her gallbladder diet, she surrounded herself with love.

In three weeks, her gallbladder attacks subsided and disappeared. As a result, surgery was canceled.

A year later Indiana sent me an amusing postcard from Venice where she goes every October to write. Her card said that she and her gallbladder felt very loved, and both adored the Italian food. Since then, it's been four years. Indiana's gallbladder is still fine.

Many factors contributed to her physical and emotional healing. To restore her emotional health, Indiana had to discover that she was creating her sense of betrayal. While her sons were leaving to go off to school, they were not betraying her.

While it was likely their pending departure was retriggering an earlier time when Indiana was betrayed, we did not explore what that may have been. We certainly could have, but didn't since her condition improved so easily.

Once she stopped creating the negative emotions of betrayal, she could give herself the love she needed to heal emotionally. It's likely this shift in emotions also influenced her physical recovery.

Truth Is Evolving

As you listen to your inner wisdom, you'll discover that truth is not fixed. It is alive and evolving. What may be true now may be but a half-truth tomorrow.

As you attune to your inner knowing, you'll realize it always tells you the next truth as it emerges.

Welcome your truths, remembering the excerpt from the poem by Earl Balfour, the English philosopher and statesman, who was Prime Minister from 1902-1905:

> Our highest truths are but half truths;
> Think not to settle down forever in any truth.
> Make use of it as a tent in which
> to pass the summer night,
> But build no house of it or it will be your tomb.

Summary

Step 2
Visualize Your Healing

1. Before and after surgery, visualize and feel in your heart, mind and being your ideal surgical outcome. Make your imagery come alive, using all of your senses — seeing, feeling, smelling and touching. This is very different from having a two-dimensional picture in your mind.

2. Focus on the healed outcome of your operation rather than on the surgical process of getting there. Ask your surgeon to describe and even draw a picture of it.

3. When worries about your operation pop into your mind, switch them to pictures of your healed result, as if you were changing the channel on a TV. By repeatedly visualizing the positive, healed image, there will soon come a time when you will believe it. It is a kind of gentle surrender that allows healing rather than commanding it.

4. In the days or weeks before surgery, visualizing your healed end-result calms you. Some people have found it also improved their physical condition.

5. Talk to the part of your body having surgery, asking what comforting emotion does it want you to give it, using the Relaxation CD, meditation or self-hypnosis. Once calm, let an image appear of the part of your body that needs healing.

6. Even if you don't see a picture, be still and open yourself to the answers to the five questions below. You may hear a voice that is similar to your intuition or have a sense of inner knowing. Most of all, trust yourself and your inner knowing.

Ask the part of your body:

* "What comforting feeling do you want me to give you?"
* "What color is the feeling?"
* "How many times a day do you want me to give you this feeling?"
* "During each healing session, how many minutes do you want to experience this comforting feeling?"
* "Is there anything else you want to tell me?"

7. When you envision your healing, feel as well as see the comforting feeling flow through and bathe the part of your body that is healing.

8. It's better to visualize your healing process for five minutes, four times a day, rather than 20 minutes once a day.

9. Every image, thought and feeling is a visualization. If you imagine a positive outcome for 20 minutes and then worry about your health for the rest of the day, your worry will obviously cancel out your positive imagery.

10. The CD guides you through visualizing three end-results:

* For the first end-result, be in your hospital room after surgery. Hear a friend, family member or a nurse asking, "How do you feel?" You say, "I feel comfortable."

* For the second end-result, imagine doing something you love to do that means you are recovering well. See, hear, smell and feel all your sensations.

* For the third end-result, enjoy being fully recovered doing something you love to do with someone you love. You might be taking a walk, having dinner or dancing.

11. Visualize your healed outcome for one minute throughout the day as you wait for an elevator, a red traffic light or while you wash the dishes.

12. If your doctor has prescribed medication, do you imagine the healing qualities of the pills or wince as you swallow them, afraid of negative side effects?

13. How long do you believe it will take to heal? Do you believe you deserve to recover easily? Ask your surgeon for the names of people to talk to who have had good recoveries.

14. Add your ideas here:

Step 3

Organize
a Support Group

> ...the quality of our relationships may have more to do with how often we get sick and how soon we get well than our genes, chemistry, diet or environment.
>
> — Bruce Larson

The emotional support you receive from your family and friends strengthens your immune system, boosting your recovery. Here are strategies to focus the love of your closest relationships before and after surgery.

When friends say, "How can I help?" Ask them to send you peace, tranquility or love for the half-hour before your operation. Decide which emotion will comfort you the most. For some it's love, for others it is peace or tranquility.

When Martha Jacoby of Belmont, Massachusetts, was facing surgery, she asked friends to wrap her in a "pink blanket of love" for half an hour before her operation. She said, "I felt a blanket of love tucked around me from my head to my toes, as I lay on a gurney in the hallway outside the operating room. As I looked at the clock, it was 9 a.m., just the time I had asked friends to send me love. I felt so peaceful."

When Frank Urbanowski, of Cambridge, Massachusetts, was getting ready for surgery, he asked his Zen meditation group to wrap him in a "purple, down-filled comforter of love." After surgery, he said, "I felt the love all around me as I waited for my operation."

When you tell friends the emotion you want to feel, express it in a colorful picture. Saying "wrap me in a pink blanket of love" conjures up a more vivid image than merely saying "send me love."

Your three-dimensional picture makes the emotion come alive. As a result, your friends' visualizations will be imbued with more feeling, creating a stronger emotion that you will feel.

How Many People Do You Need?
Two or three friends are plenty. People who know how to focus their hearts and minds can easily envelop you in peace. But don't limit yourself. If you

have six or eight friends or a prayer group that wants to send you peace, let them all do it. The more people, the stronger the feeling that you will experience. Some friends will want to wrap you in love for the entire operation.

Set up a free blog at www.CaringBridge.org as a way to ask friends and family to wrap you in your Blanket of Love. It gives everyone a way to send you emails of love and support before and after surgery. And you can send daily updates on your recovery. This blog creates your private bubble of support.

How to Project an Emotion

While some friends will be familiar with sending you an emotion, others may ask, "How do I do this?" Tell them, "Let your mind go back to a time you felt a lot of love for me. Replay that scene in your mind until you feel the love. When you feel connected to me, as if I were right next to you, wrap me in a pink Blanket of Love for 30 minutes, starting at ___ o'clock."

Specify the half-hour before your surgery. Choose the color of the blanket that feels right for you. Even if surgery is delayed, you'll be comforted by the love or peace that already surrounds you.

The key to projecting an emotion to another is feeling connected to that person while you send it. It's similar to being in love, feeling bonded to the other, even when you are not with him or her.

It's this kind of linking you want to experience. It doesn't mean you have to be in love with the person. It just means that having a sense of connectedness allows the emotion to be felt by the other.

Letting your mind go back to a time you felt a lot of love for the person often creates this bonded sensation. While the person may be waiting for surgery in another room, another city or another country, you can easily envelop him or her in peace — or love.

Peaceful Support Group

An anxious spouse and friends will discover that sending you love will also comfort them at a time they are worried about you. In fact, you'll want the people who will be with you before and after your operation to feel peaceful because their emotional states will affect you.

If your significant other or friends are hovering anxiously around your hospital bed or sitting beside you in a waiting area, you'll feel their fear. If you let it, their unspoken fear can make you afraid.

Similarly, if your support persons have learned to relax, their peace will comfort you during the half-hour or several hours of waiting before surgery.

If your primary support persons do not know how to relax, ask them if they would like to use the

Relaxation CD. If so, have them to read Step 1: Relax to Feel Peaceful, which explains how to use the CD. With daily practice, they will be able to count themselves into a deep state of relaxation which will complement your own.

While I'm sure you know how much other people's moods can affect you when you are in the same room, you may be wondering how their emotions can influence you when they are not in your physical presence. Although it is not understood how it happens, more than 100 studies document that it does occur.

An overview of the research is presented in *Healing Words* by Dr. Larry Dossey, an internist and former Chief of Staff of Medical City Dallas Hospital in Texas.

Prayers Reduced the Need for Antibiotics

Further evidence is provided by Dr. Randolph Byrd, a cardiologist at San Francisco General Hospital. His research showed that 192 patients who were prayed for were five times less likely to require antibiotics and three times less likely to develop pulmonary edema, a condition in which the lungs fill with fluid when the heart fails to pump properly.

In addition, those receiving daily prayers were less likely to require endotracheal intubation, meaning a tube is inserted into patients' throats and attached to a mechanical ventilator that breathes for them. None of the group receiving prayers required ventilatory support, while 12 of the control group needed it.

To control for influencing factors, a computer randomly assigned the 393 patients to either the group receiving prayers or the control group receiving no prayers. Neither the patients nor doctors knew to which group the patients were assigned. Prayer groups prayed daily for the patients, knowing only their first names.[1]

The results of Dr. Byrd's study are remarkable. If a drug study had these results, it would be hailed, becoming the drug of choice.

Support Person before Surgery

In addition to having your friends send you love before surgery, also arrange for your spouse or closest friend to be with you until you go into the operating room. Otherwise your spouse may be sitting in a nearby waiting room while you are left alone in a holding-area before surgery. With advance permission, your spouse could be with you.

If requested, your surgeon can often make these arrangements. If not, your doctor can tell you who to call at the hospital. Hospitals are eager to meet your individual needs as a consumer; you'll find them very cooperative.

The benefits of preoperative emotional support have been documented by three studies at the Rigshospitalet in Copenhagen, Denmark. The research showed that patients' anxiety was less when a member of the anesthesiology department was with them before and after surgery. Their anxiety was much less than that of patients in the control group, who had tranquilizers rather than the support of a person.[2]

Because hospitals need to contain costs, it's unlikely yours will provide a staff member to be with you. However, you can organize this service by having a spouse or close friend at your side.

Emotional Support during Labor
In a controlled study in a hospital affiliated with Baylor College of Medicine in Houston, Texas, women in labor had 56% fewer caesarean sections when they had the ongoing emotional support of a doula, a woman trained to assist in the hours of labor prior to birth.

Labors were shortened by two hours when compared to the control group. Half as many babies required long hospitalizations after birth.[3]

Intensive Care Unit

If you will be in the intensive care unit, arrange permission for your spouse and friends to stay with you longer than the 10 to 20 minutes usually allowed for each visit. Most nurses will agree to your request depending on your condition.

Although only one person can be with you at a time, you can orchestrate a relay of friends who will surround you with love during their short stays. Their caring will gently enfold you as they come and go throughout the day and night.

Calming My Fears

I remember having to calm my fears before my grandmother, Peggy Dickson Friar of Haverford, Pennsylvania, had surgery. I felt frightened as I walked along the hallway to her room in the Bryn Mawr Hospital. The smells of the hospital brought back my childhood fears of having my tonsils and appendix removed in the same hospital.

Within several hours, my grandmother was scheduled to have a mastectomy. She was worried even though her doctor reassured her that at age 83 her body's metabolism was so slowed down that she might outlive a recurrence of cancer.

Knowing that my anxiety would only make my grandmother feel worse, to calm myself, I leaned against the wall outside her doorway. As I counted myself into a deep state of relaxation, the tension and fear drained from my body.

After a few minutes of deep relaxation, I let my mind go back to a time I had felt a loving connection with my grandmother, feeling my love flowing out to her and hers flowing back to me. Centered in love, I opened the door.

The nurse had just taken my grandmother's blood pressure. It was so dangerously high the operation needed to be delayed. The nurse said she would be back in 20 minutes to check the blood pressure.

As I sat beside my grandmother's hospital bed, I remembered all the times her love had helped me through difficult situations. I held her hand as we talked.

All the while, I focused my attention on my heart, feeling my love flowing to her. Whenever I slid back into my fears, I drew my awareness to my heart, feeling my love for her.

When the nurse returned, she looked surprised, finding that the blood pressure reading had dropped to normal. She turned to me, smiling and said, "Whatever you are doing, just continue. Her blood pressure is fine. It's safe to go ahead with the operation."

Your Support Group

Open yourself to receive all the ways your community of friends reaches out to you through their useful information, concerns and kindnesses. Talking about your health problem often reduces your fears. The song by The Beatles is right: "I get by with a little help from my friends."

Your friends who give you emotional support also benefit. Research shows that people involved in helping others through community activities live longer. In a study of 2,700 residents in Tecumseh, Michigan, men who did volunteer work were two and a half times less likely to die of all causes of disease than their non-volunteering peers.[4]

Ask for Practical Help

Make a list of the specific ways you want to be helped before and after your operation. If you have young children at home, ask your sister or a good friend to stay at your house to take care of your children while you are in the hospital.

If you have a spouse or a significant other, this will give them more time to be with you. Without a friend running your household, your spouse will become a wreck, racing back and forth between you in the hospital and the kids at home.

If you don't have a family that needs care, you may need a friend to feed your cat, water your plants and collect your mail. Several friends can take turns bringing you home-cooked meals. You'll probably want one or two close friends to be with you in the hospital before and after surgery.

When people ask "How can I help?" match up that person with an item on your list that suits them. If your children have never loved your sister, and your sister insists on taking care of them, diplomatically thank her, and find a friend your children feel closer to. Find some other way that your sister can help. Maybe she is a good organizer. If so, she can do the follow-up to make sure each friend carries out the ways you want to be helped.

When Others Are Not Supportive

Don't be surprised if one friend pulls away because he or she can't cope with you having an operation. Although you may feel hurt by their withdrawal, don't take it personally. It only means this person has unresolved issues with illness or hospitals that are triggered by your situation. While one friend may pull away, many more will draw closer to you.

If you come from a family that is not supportive, you may find that your need for emotional support sadly highlights how emotionally unavailable your family has always been.

For instance, when Carol Andrews of Seattle was preparing for cataract surgery, her mother forgot that she was having surgery. Carol said, "Her forgetting reminded me of how alone I was as a child. My mother was always self-absorbed. If it wasn't happening to her, it wasn't happening at all."

If your mother or another important person in your life is emotionally withdrawn, don't give them the role of your primary support person who goes through surgery with you. You'll only be painfully disappointed, feeling their coldness at a time you need love.

Break Your Pattern of Isolation

If your way of dealing with an emotionally unavailable family is to be independent, do it yourself and never ask them for help, use this situation as an opportunity to break your pattern of isolation. Ask for support.

You'll probably feel vulnerable or scared the first times you risk asking for what you need. This may be the vulnerability you felt as a child when you needed help and felt the emptiness of no one responding to you. It caused the ache of feeling unloved — of being alone.

Now, when you find that your requests call forth your friends' love and assistance, it gets easier to ask the next time.

If you have always been the person who takes care of everyone else, you'll need to let others take care of you. If you have the habit of putting other people's needs before your own, this is a time to give yourself permission to put your needs first.

Ask a nurturing friend to be your support person. He or she can be with you through the hospital check-in process, hold your hand while you wait for surgery and comfort you when you come out of the recovery room. If necessary, your friend can be your medical advocate, using his or her voice and energy to arrange for any special medical needs that may arise.

For example, if you are uncomfortable, a friend can quickly get a nurse to assist you. Because of cutbacks in health care, the nursing staff is smaller and less able to respond to your needs as fast. If a friend gets the attention of a nurse, you're likely to get help sooner. And if you are scheduled for medical tests, it's reassuring to have a friend check that you are getting the tests your doctor ordered.

Healing Power of Families

Some hospitals make it easy for your spouse or friend to spend the night in your room. If you would like to arrange this comfort, ask for it. Nurses have observed that patients who have the love of friends and family often recover faster than patients without someone who loves them.

For example, in the Philippines when someone is in the hospital, the whole family rallies around. It's a time of reconciliation. Brothers who have not spoken for years are reunited. Grudges and resentments are dropped, replaced with love for the patient.

Family members do all the care and bathing of the patient. They even provide the meals. Nurses only give the medication. A couch is provided in each room so that a family member has a place to sleep next to the patient.

Healing in Hispanic Communities

The healing power of families is also seen in Hispanic communities. In *Natural Health, Natural Medicine,* Dr. Andrew T. Weil, writes:

> A nurse at the University of Arizona medical center told me that she worked for a number of years in the pediatric intensive care unit. During her time there she saw twelve children recover miraculously from apparently fatal head injuries. They had been in bicycle or motorbike accidents, were in deepest coma, had flat EEGs (brain-wave patterns), and were given up for dead by the attending physicians.

> She saw twelve children in that extreme state come back to full consciousness and life, to the amazement of their doctors. What caught her attention most was that all of the children were Hispanic.

In her words, "I've never seen an Anglo kid recover from such an injury. And do you know what the difference is? When a Hispanic kid is in a coma like that, the whole family is around the bed day and night, talking to him, praying for him, loving him. The Anglo kids are there all by themselves, unconscious children in beds in intensive care, all alone."

We are not meant to be all alone. We are meant to be parts of bigger families, bands, tribes. Don't settle for nuclear family contraction. Extend!

Ask Questions

Don't be shy about asking questions. The hospital staff welcomes your questions, knowing that patients who are involved in their medical care often get well sooner than patients who passively accept what's done to them.

To safeguard yourself, double check your medication. Ask if the red pill you are about to swallow is the medication your doctor prescribed. The name may be printed on the tablet. If not, request the name and dosage of the pill.

Nurses will be glad you are asking, knowing that the more you are involved in your care at the hospital, the more you'll be responsible for your care at home.

Ways of Being Together

In the hospital and at home, find ways of being with your family and friends that are the most healing. If talking tires you, say so.

Discover the ways of being together that are beyond words. Feel what would comfort you and ask for it. Maybe you want someone to hold your hand, stroke your forehead or just sit quietly beside you. When a friend is with you, ask him or her to wrap you in love. You'll feel loved — and so will they.

Meditation

Meditation is another nonverbal way of being together. If you and your spouse meditate, it's very peaceful to do it together in your hospital room or at home.

Hugs Release Endorphins

Also, there will be times you feel like being hugged. Ask for it. A hug is powerful medicine. This expression of affection triggers the release of endorphins, chemical substances in your brain that make you feel good. And if you are having pain, endorphins are known to lessen it.

Unconscious Patients

Even if people are unconscious, experiences show they often feel loved by their family who gather around their bed. For example, when the late Perky Lloyd's close friend, Mia, was unconscious in the

Bryn Mawr Hospital, Perky called me saying, "I feel so helpless. I'm sitting on one side of Mia's bed and her husband is on the other. Is there anything more I can do?"

I told her there was a lot more. First, she needed to meditate to become centered. When her mind was quiet, I suggested she remember a time she had experienced a close, loving feeling with Mia. Perky said, "We've been friends for year, I remember lots of them."

A few hours later Perky called me saying, "It's wonderful. Whenever I feel my love for Mia, she squeezes my hand. Her doctors say she is unconscious but she must be feeling something."

Massage

If you have friends who are trained in massage or one of the many hands-on healing methods, let their hands do their work, when you feel ready to be touched. Even if they do not have specific training, their touch will still be a loving one. It is the love that heals.

The calming benefits of massage were shown in a recent study at the University of Miami School of Medicine by Dr. Tiffany Fields. Children receiving massages had lower levels of the stress hormone cortisol when compared with the children in the control group.[5]

A caring touch can be effective anywhere on the body. For example, when Jack Mommer was recovering from surgery at the Mayo Clinic, his head, torso and arms were so covered by bandages and monitors, his feet were the only place he could be touched. His wife, Mary, and his sister, Billie Lee, took turns massaging his feet. Jack found it soothing. And they were relieved there was something they could do to help.

Therapeutic Touch

In America, more than 100,000 nurses have been trained in Therapeutic Touch (TT). It is a healing method developed in 1972 by Dr. Dolores Krieger, professor of nursing at New York University and Dora Kunz. Without touching the body, practitioners use their hands to influence the field of energy that pulsates in and around the physical body.

Physicists call this energy a force field. A growing body of clinical research shows that Therapeutic Touch lowers blood pressure, reduces pain and helps wounds heal faster.

At the University of Missouri, nurses Virginia Bzdek and Elizabeth Keller found that patients' tension headaches were eased for as long as four hours after a five-minute session of TT.[6]

If you would like to experience the calming and healing effect of this treatment, ask which nurses in the hospital are trained in TT. You may even find you have several friends who have taken courses in this method.

Courses in Therapeutic Touch are given in more than 12 medical schools and 80 colleges and universities in America. To find a practitioner, see the Resources section on page 234.

Reiki

Reiki (pronounced ray-key) is another method of hands-on healing. Its an ancient practice described in Buddhist texts as healing the body using universal energy. Trained practitioners channel energy through their hands which are placed on your body.

You can also give energy to yourself. While Reiki classes will teach you the methodology, experiment by putting your hands on a part of your body that needs healing. By having the clear intention to let universal energy flow through your hands, they may become warm, or perhaps tingle, as the energy moves through your hands into your body.

To find a Reiki Master, a person trained to give a healing session or take a class to learn how to give it to yourself and others, see page 235 in Resources. Each Reiki Master is different. Have sessions with several until you find the ones you like.

Hands-On Healing in the Operating Room

At New York-Presbyterian Hospital/Columbia in New York, Dr. Mehmet Oz, a cardiothoracic surgeon, has experimented with having two people giving hands-on healing to the patient while he performs heart surgery. He finds it comforts patients and appears to speed healing.

Beware of People Who Drain You

While you feel energized by some friends, have you ever been drained by others? Avoid these people while you are healing. They may be well meaning, but they are energy vampires.

If they want to visit, they will only tire you at a time you need all your energy for your recovery. Postpone seeing them until you are well.

If you can't avoid close relatives or business associates who drain you, at least find some way to shorten their visit. Tell them by phone that you need to limit their stay to 15 minutes. You can always explain that you need to rest.

Healing Power of Pets

When Carolyn Ellis of Weston, Massachusetts, was recuperating from surgery, she curled up in bed with her favorite cat, Paganini. She called it "my pet therapy." Whenever she felt tired, she took a nap with Paganini nestled beside her.

If you have a favorite pet, let the comfort of this animal be with you while you recover at home. Feeling a pet's love soothes you, stimulating your parasympathetic nervous system which speeds healing.

When 45 women had their own dogs at their side, there was a reduction in their levels of stress when measured by psychologists Drs. Karen Allen and James Blascovich at the State University of New York.

Some Hospitals Allow Pets
A few hospitals already recognize the healing power of pets. Some hospital administrators encourage adults and children to have their own dog or cat in their room, knowing that research shows people heal faster when they have a pet with them. A small number of hospitals even have "loaner dogs" for patients who would like one.

The Delta Society, an international non-profit organization, trains and certifies owners and their pets to visit people in homes and hospitals.

If you would like a visit from a pet, a cat, dog or even a rabbit, call the headquarters in Bellevue, Washington: (425) 679-5500; www.DeltaSociety.org.

My Hope

My hope is that the stories of the healing power of your family, friends, pets and community will inspire you to create emotional support while you are healing — and afterwards.

A strong network of friends, family and community not only helps you heal, it also protects against disease and death. This was shown in a nine-year study of 7,000 residents of Alameda County in California. Those who did not have many close friends or relatives died at a rate two to five times greater than those with strong social ties.[7]

Because Western societies are becoming more fragmented, you'll consciously need to create your community.

Summary

Step 3
Organize a Support Group

1. Ask friends and family to send you peace, tranquility or love for the half-hour before your operation.

2. Ask each person to visualize a colorful, three-dimensional image, such as wrapping you in a pink blanket of love.

3. If friends ask how to send you love, tell them, "Let your mind go back to a time you felt a lot of love for me. Replay that scene in your mind until you feel the love welling up in your heart. Then for half an hour, as your love flows to me, wrap me in a pink blanket of it."

4. The key to projecting an emotion to another person is feeling fused or connected to that person while you are sending it.

5. More than 100 research studies have documented that people's emotions can affect another person not in their physical presence.

6. A remarkable study by Dr. Randolph Byrd, a cardiologist at San Francisco General Hospital, showed that 192 patients who were prayed for were

five times less likely to require antibiotics than the 201 patients in the control group.

7. If your primary support persons do not know how to relax, ask if they would like to develop the skill. Offer them the use of the Relaxation CD.

8. For your emotional support, ask your surgeon how to arrange permission for your closest friend and/or spouse to be with you right up until you go into the operating room. Hospital staff members are eager to meet your individual needs as a consumer.

9. Medical studies show that the emotional support you receive from your network of family and friends strengthens your immune system, facilitating your recovery.

10. If you will be in the intensive care unit following surgery, arrange special permission for your spouse and friends to stay with you longer than the 10 or 30 minutes usually allowed for each visit. Although only one person can be with you at a time, you can orchestrate a relay of friends who each surround you in love.

11. The hospital staff welcomes your questions, knowing that patients who are involved in their medical care often get well sooner than patients who passively accept what's done to them.

12. Find the ways of being with your family and friends that are the most healing for you. If talking tires you, say so. Ask, if you want someone to hold your hand, stroke your forehead or just sit quietly beside you.

13. Allow friends trained in massage or one of the many hands-on healing techniques to do their work.

14. In some hospitals, some nurses are trained in Therapeutic Touch (TT). It is a healing method developed in 1972 by Dr. Dolores Kreiger, professor of nursing at New York University and Dora Kunz. Without touching the body, practitioners use their hands to influence the field of energy that pulsates in and around the physical body. TT lowers blood pressure, reduces pain and helps wounds heal faster.

15. While healing, avoid the people who drain you.

16. Some hospitals recognize the healing power of pets. A pet's love soothes you and stimulates your parasympathetic nervous system, creating the chemicals that boost your immune system, speeding healing.

17. Add your ideas here:

Step 4

Use
Healing Statements

> ... the patients who were exposed to positive
> suggestions showed a reduction of 23% in
> their morphine requirements in the first
> 24 hours postoperatively.
>
> — T.T.C. McLintock

Research from around the world shows that —
contrary to what has been commonly believed
— when you are anesthetized and unconscious, you
hear what is said during surgery. Furthermore, you
are powerfully influenced by what you hear, much like
a person under hypnosis.

For example, studies at Beth Israel Medical
Center in New York, Emory University School of
Medicine in Atlanta, St. Thomas's Hospital in
London and the Royal Infirmary in Glasgow all show

that patients who had positive statements spoken to them during general anesthesia recovered more quickly with less pain and complications than the patients in the control group, who were not given the statements.[1-4]

The implications of the research are remarkable: Having your doctor or a nurse say specific healing statements to you during your operation can directly affect how much pain medication you take and how long it takes you to heal.

If you will be awake during surgery, having local or regional anesthesia, you'll want your doctor or nurse to say the therapeutic statements. By using the Relaxation CD to put yourself in a deep state of relaxation during surgery, you will be highly suggestible. As a result, your recovery will require less pain medication and you will heal faster.

Therapeutic statements may someday be a routine procedure. Until then, you need to ask your doctor to say them. It is your legal right.

Your surgeon and anesthesiologist may already use therapeutic statements. If not, you're probably wondering: Why aren't doctors more sensitive to the powerful effect of their words and actions?

Since the first public demonstration of anesthesia in 1846 at Harvard Medical School, most doctors were taught that a well-anesthetized patient cannot hear anything said in the operating room. This assumption is no longer believed to be true. Research shows that the conversations and comments in the operating room are registered in your unconscious mind, even if you do not consciously recall them following surgery.

While there is ongoing scientific debate about exactly how much an anesthetized patient can hear, one point is clear: **You never stop hearing.**

During general anesthesia, auditory stimuli are registered in the cerebral cortex. As anesthesia is increased most brain areas become depressed, but the auditory system remains functional.

There is even evidence that people in a coma can hear. It is now common practice for loved ones to sit by the bed and talk to and hold the hand of someone in a coma. When they regain consciousness, patients often recount how they heard the conversations and felt the loving presence of their family while they were unconscious. The loving words or the friendly lick of a favorite dog have been known to be the stimulation that brings people back to consciousness.

However, until this growing body of evidence is more widely known and taught in medical schools, you have to take the initiative and ask your doctor to use the positive statements.

Remember, it is your body and your well-being. It is up to you to seize the moment and make the most of this opportunity to influence your healing.

Because more patients are taking an active role in their healing, doctors are growing accustomed to requests of this type. Many encourage your requests, knowing that the more you are involved, the more likely you both are to create a healthy doctor-patient partnership that will speed your recovery.

In my 18 years of teaching thousands of people how to ask their doctors to use the statements, all the doctors welcomed their patients' requests. As a result, many people have found their rapport with their doctors increased as they discovered how open their physicians were to their ideas. Ideally, you should feel comfortable talking with your doctor about anything you believe may help you.

Brief History of Research
To better understand the concept of healing statements, here is an overview of some of the studies showing their benefits.

As early as the 1950s, Dr. David B. Cheek, a gynecologist in California, researched and published his findings of how his patients were traumatized by their doctors' negative remarks in the operating room. He cautioned surgeons against having damaging conversations in the presence of unconscious patients.[5]

Influenced by Dr. Cheek's research, Dr. L. S. Wolfe and Dr. J. B. Millet of Ithaca, New York, in 1959 gave 1,500 patients intraoperative suggestions that they would heal well and feel comfortable after their operations. Their findings showed that 70% of the adults and 100% of the children in the study needed no pain medication at all after surgery.

Although they did not have a control group, Drs. Wolfe and Millet found the results remarkable when compared with the usual medical outcome. In fact, nurses at the hospital were so impressed with the results, finding it much easier to administer postoperative care, that they encouraged other physicians to "talk" to their patients during surgery.[6]

In 1959 Dr. Donald D. Hutchings, an anesthesiologist in Bath, New York, conducted a similar study with 200 patients. In the small, 75 bed hospital where Dr. Hutchings practiced, he repeated the same positive statements to all his patients while they were anesthetized: "You will heal promptly and well. You will awaken from the anesthetic as if you had been asleep at night, feeling rested and refreshed. You will have no pain at the place that was operated on. You will eat well and sleep well, enjoying your hospital stay. You will urinate easily and move your bowels regularly."

The results showed that 70% of the adults required no pain medication following surgery. Although there was no control group, Dr. Hutchings observed, "Postoperative care was made easier. Patients were more comfortable and more cooperative and healing was hastened." As a result, he urged other anesthesiologists to conduct similar studies.[7]

Landmark Study by Dr. Levinson

In 1965 Dr. Bernard Levinson, a psychiatrist in South Africa, conducted a study exploring the effect of doctors' words on surgical patients. His research was greatly influenced by his own experiences when he was a Resident Anesthetist in a Chelsea Hospital in London in 1953.

There he had vividly witnessed "that every time there was a crisis in the operating theater a current of anxiety flowed between the surgeon and myself, [the anesthetist], via the patient...On these occasions I could almost watch the anxiety creep [from the surgeon] along the patient's body to my end of the operation."

Inspired by his personal experiences in the operating room and the work of Dr. Cheek, Dr. Levinson designed what was to become a landmark study. He staged a mock "crisis" in the middle of 10 operations.

When each patient had reached an extremely deep level of anesthesia, called Stage III, as shown by an electroencephalogram (EEG), an instrument that measures brain-wave activity, he dramatically said, "Stop the operation. I don't like the patient's color. The lips are turning too blue. I'm going to give a little oxygen." Then he would pump the rebreathing bag and loudly say, "There. That's better now. You can carry on with the operation."

At the time of his study, no one in the operating room believed that an unconscious patient could hear. A month after the 10 patients were discharged from the hospital, Dr. Levinson met with each of them and used hypnosis to discover what they recalled from the operation.

Although none of the patients had a conscious memory of the "crisis," under hypnosis, four patients recalled verbatim everything that had been said in the operating room. They even knew which doctor had been talking and where they were standing in the room at the time of the "crisis." Four other patients had partial recall and became extremely anxious while being regressed back to the event. The other two patients had no recall.

Dr. Levinson's ground-breaking study clearly demonstrated that even deeply anesthetized patients can hear what is said in the operating theater.[8]

St. Thomas's Hospital in London

In 1988 at St. Thomas's Hospital in London, Dr. Carlton Evans and Dr. H.P. Richardson gave therapeutic suggestions to women undergoing total abdominal hysterectomies. Of the 39 women in the double-blind study, half the group heard a tape recording during surgery saying, "How quickly you recover from your operation depends upon you — the more you relax, the more comfortable you will be. You will not feel sick, you will not have any pain. The operation seems to be going very well, and the patient is fine."

Their findings showed that the women who heard the positive suggestions recovered more quickly, had fewer complications, and left the hospital sooner than the control group.[9]

Royal Infirmary in Glasgow

In 1990 at the Royal Infirmary in Glasgow, Scotland, Dr. T. T. C. McLintock and his research team conducted a similar study with 30 women having total abdominal hysterectomies. During surgery the women heard a recording stating, "You will feel warm and comfortable, calm and relaxed; any pain that you feel after the operation will not concern you."

The patients receiving these suggestions used 23% less morphine on the day of surgery than the control group.[10]

Emory University School of Medicine

In 1992 Marcia Steinberg, a nurse anesthetist, and Dr. Allen Hord, an anesthesiologist, both at Emory University School of Medicine in Atlanta, conducted a study to refute or corroborate the Scottish findings. Their research showed that 30 patients, chosen at random to hear positive suggestions during surgery, used less pain medication than the control group on the first day following surgery.[11]

Yale-New Haven Hospital

Dr. Bernie S. Siegel, a former surgeon at Yale-New Haven Hospital in New Haven, Connecticut and best-selling author of *Love, Medicine and Miracles*, routinely conveyed messages of hope and healing to his patients during surgery. He writes, "I keep talking to patients throughout the operation, telling them how things are progressing and enlisting their cooperation if I need it."

"For example, I may suggest that they stop bleeding or lower their blood pressure or pulse. People who have worked with me in the operating room know how effective these suggestions can be. Often when a patient's pulse rate is too high during an operation, I'll simply say, We'd like your pulse to be eighty-six.' I always pick a specific number because I want everyone to see the pulse go down to that exact number."

"Beached Whale"

There are also many anecdotal case reports in the anesthesiology literature about patients' recoveries being negatively effected because someone in the operating room made an insulting remark about the patient, when the patient was unconscious during surgery. For example, a woman's recovery from surgery was greatly impaired until she remembered that during her operation her surgeon had called her a "beached whale" in reference to her excess weight.

To verify it, her nurse checked with a nurse who had been in the operating room during the patient's surgery. The nurse confirmed that the disparaging comment had indeed been made by the doctor. Although the patient had been unconscious, she recalled the offensive remark, which appeared to have slowed her postoperative recovery.[12]

Innocent Remarks

Even an innocent remark by your doctor can have a negative effect. When you are having surgery, you are in a mental state of extreme alertness whether you are unconscious or conscious. You are very alert because you are concerned about your survival.

As a result, you interpret information differently than you would in your normal, everyday state of mind. In an alert state, information that would ordinarily be neutral to you is often interpreted negatively.

For example, your surgeon might say, "It's all over," meaning the operation is finished. But you could interpret the remark to mean: "It's hopeless. There is nothing more the doctors can do." In another situation, the surgeon's comment, "It's no good. It's got a hole in it," could refer to a hole in one of the surgical gloves. However, you could interpret the surgeon's statement to mean that the part of your body being operated on is "no good" and "has a hole in it."

Erasmus University in Rotterdam

Situations, as well was words, can also be misinterpreted. Dr. Benno Bonke, a psychologist at Erasmus University in Rotterdam in the Netherlands, tells a story that demonstrates this point. Dr. Bonke and his Dutch colleagues have done extensive research and writing about the psychological consequences of awareness in so-called unconscious patients.

While a patient was regaining consciousness in the recovery room, a nurse noticed that dust from repair work on the ceiling was falling on the patient's face. To protect him, she pulled a sheet over his head. As the anesthesia began to wear off, the patient started to wake up. He was frightened to find a sheet covering his head. To him, it meant that he must have died and was in the morgue. The scare did not help his recovery.

Routine Use of Healing Statements

When Dr. Monica Furlong, an anesthesiologis, was at Beth Israel Medical Center in New York City, she often used healing suggestions in surgery. She recalled a typical operating room scene where one of the doctors assisting in a chemical face peel, a type of cosmetic surgery that removes a layer of skin to reveal the less-wrinkled skin beneath, loudly remarked, "That's really going to hurt during recovery."

Hoping to counteract the effect of the negative suggestion, Dr. Furlong leaned down and began talking into her patient's ear, saying over and over, "Following this operation, your face will feel warm and tingling and comfortable."

An hour later when Dr. Furlong saw her patient regaining consciousness in the recovery room, she walked over and asked her, "How does your face feel?" Her patient turned to her and said, "My face feels warm and tingling and comfortable." Clearly, this patient, had registered the therapeutic suggestion.

Based on the principle that patients hear all the time, from the induction of the anesthesia to the end of the operation, Dr. Furlong makes it a practice to talk to her patients throughout surgery, telling them what she is doing and how it will help them.

For example, she says, "I am spraying your throat. The spray will be cool and soothing. It has medicines to protect your throat." When she inserts a trachea tube, she says, "I am putting a tube in your throat to help your breathing. This tube is here to protect you."

Several times during an operation, it is natural for her to say other positive suggestions, such as, "The operation is going very well. You will wake up feeling calm and relaxed. You will heal quickly and comfortably. You will wake up feeling thirsty and hungry."

50% Less Pain Medication

Since so many of her patients appeared to benefit from her statements during surgery, Dr. Furlong designed a study to document her observations. Her research findings showed that patients who heard therapeutic statements played on a tape during surgery used 50% less pain medication on the day of surgery as compared to the patients in the control group, who heard a blank tape recording.[13]

Dr. Furlong presented her findings in 1989 at the First International Symposium in Memory and Awareness at the University of Glasgow in Scotland, where more than 100 anesthesiologists and psychologists from 21 countries met to discuss their research.

In April 1992, a second symposium was sponsored by Emory University School of Medicine in Atlanta, Georgia. In June 1995 a third symposium was held in the Netherlands. It was organized by the Faculty of Medicine and Health Sciences of Erasmus University in Rotterdam.

From those conferences and other studies, a highly significant body of research demonstrates that words spoken during surgery can affect a patient's recovery, positively or negatively.

Healing Statements

While there is more to be learned about why therapeutic statements are so effective, there is no doubt that you can benefit by using them. Doctors are extremely receptive to your request to have therapeutic statements spoken during your operation, even though it may not yet be part of the procedure.

At the Mayo Clinic, when Jack Mommer gave the Healing Statements to his anesthesiologist, Dr. Peggy Wagoner, she said, "I am glad to say these as you go under the anesthesia. Other patients often make the same request."

It is your legal right to have the Healing Statements said to you during surgery. Your right to make a reasonable request regarding your care is given to you in every hospital's Patient's Bill of Rights.

At Brigham and Women's Hospital, one of the Harvard Medical School teaching hospitals, Dr. Susan L. Troyan, who specializes in breast surgery, says, "In the operating room, whether patients are conscious or unconscious, I am always reassuring them that the operation is going well."

"Sometimes a patient will give me a prayer to read out loud during surgery. Once a patient, who wanted to stop smoking, asked me to say. 'You hate cigarettes' while she was unconscious.

Asking a Doctor to Use Healing Statements

If your surgeon does not use therapeutic statements, here is how to request that your doctor use them for you. After your surgeon has answered all your questions, explain that you have read about the benefits of positive statements spoken during surgery.

Tell your doctor, "There are four statements that I would like you or the anesthesiologist to say to me during my operation." Give your doctor a page of the Healing Statements with the blanks filled in.

Ask your surgeon if he or she would like to be the person to say them. Some surgeons like to deliver the statements themselves, while others prefer that the anesthesiologist or a nurse do it.

Even if you or your surgeon decide that the anesthesiologist will say the statements, continue telling your surgeon about them. This way your surgeon can understand and support their use. While your surgeon does not have to believe in the benefits of the statements, he or she can respect your wishes and agree to facilitate them.

Surgeons frequently say that the anesthesiologist is the best person to repeat the statements. The anesthesiologist is the doctor most attuned to your vital signs and consciousness during your operation, standing beside you, watching your face and monitoring your physiology. While your surgeon is occupied with the operation, your anesthesiologist will find it easier to lean down and say the statements or a nurse in the operating room can also say them.

First Healing Statement:

"Following this operation, you will feel comfortable and you will heal very well."

If you will be unconscious during surgery, the first Healing Statement should be repeated five times as you are going under the anesthesia.

If you will be awake during surgery and having local or regional anesthesia, it should be repeated five times as you are deeply relaxed at the beginning of surgery.

This statement gives you the suggestion to change how you experience pain. A large body of research has shown that we have a tremendous capacity to alter our sense of pain. Each person's capacity to do this is different.

If you will be unconscious during your operation, hearing the statement five times, as you go under the anesthesia, allows you to be influenced by it, again and again, as the anesthesia carries you into deeper altered states of consciousness in which you are highly suggestible.

After your operation, you may feel comfortable or you may have some discomfort or pain. It will be much less than you might have experienced had you not been told this statement.

The first statement is worded to avoid the use of the word "pain." It might seem more logical to say, "Following this operation you will have no pain and you will heal very well."

If I say, "Don't think of a pink elephant," what pops into your mind? Probably a pink elephant. It is best not to mention pain.

If You Will Be Awake during Surgery

If you will be <u>awake</u> during your operation having local or regional anesthesia, listen to the CD of the relaxation process as a way to achieve a deep state of relaxation, before, during and after surgery.

If you know the skill of self-hypnosis, it is also an excellent method to calm yourself. Deeply relaxed, you will be in an altered state in which you are highly suggestible and your recovery will benefit from the therapeutic statements.

When you are awake during an operation, there are many ways your anesthesiologist can make sure you have no discomfort. In your preoperative meeting with an anesthesiologist, you will learn about the various medical options to avoid pain. One word from you and your anesthesiologist can immediately administer medication through an IV, an intravenous tube that is put in place before surgery

Being calm during your operation allows all your muscles to relax. Otherwise, your skeletal muscles would be tensed in fear and resistance to the surgery, making the surgeon's work more difficult.

After surgery, if your muscles are relaxed, your blood circulates more easily around the incision, helping the healing process and allowing pain medication, if needed, to reach the site of surgery.

Meditation

Often I am asked, "Can I use meditation as a way to relax since I am not familiar with a relaxation process?" It is difficult to know what people experience when they meditate. If your mind wanders or you daydream, this is not meditation.

If you repeat a mantra while you meditate, be sure you can stay focused on the mantra, even if there is distracting conversation around you. If you have always meditated in the silence of a quiet room, you will not be practiced at staying centered on your mantra in a noisy room as you wait for surgery.

If you doubt your ability to meditate under stressful conditions, which can be challenging to say the least, be sure to use the Relaxation CD.

Relaxation CD

Use the CD twice a day, every day, for at least a week prior to surgery. Listening to the CD gives you the advantage of tangible words to guide you into a state of relaxation, making it easier to stay focused on the words, instead of being distracted by the conversations in the operating room.

With practice, you will be able to relax and stay relaxed, before, during and after surgery.

When Donna Beckett, a social worker in Denver, Colorado, waited for surgery, she listened to the Relaxation CD, as she lay on a gurney in a prep room at St. Joseph's Hospital-Kaiser Permanente. Her operation was set for 10 in the morning.

At 11:30 a.m. her anesthesiologist walked up to her, very apologetic about the delay, saying, "Donna, you have been waiting a long time. You're probably nervous. Let me give you a tranquilizer."

Unlike other patients who might have felt anxious, Donna was very calm, and said, "Oh no. I'm fine." After checking Donna's blood pressure, her doctor said, "It's 110/80. You are more peaceful than most tranquilizers could make you!"

Healing Statement to Reduce Bleeding

Ask your surgeon if you'll be at risk for excessive bleeding during surgery. If you are, add the following Healing Statement:

"You will have minimal bleeding during surgery." (Repeat 5 times as surgery begins.)

In addition, in the weeks prior to surgery let go of fears of bleeding by telling your body you'll have only the slightest bleeding during surgery. Affirm the statement daily until you believe it.

In a study at the University of California, Davis Medical Center, patients having orthopedic surgery of the spine had a reduction of blood loss from 900cc to 500cc, as compared to the control group, when they received preoperative suggestions.[14]

The second, third and fourth statements are each repeated five times towards the end of surgery.

Second Healing Statement:

"Your operation has gone very well."

Hearing this statement during surgery puts your mind at ease. Doctors using this statement often find their patients recover faster.

For example, Dr. Joseph T. Moskal, an orthopedic surgeon in Roanoke, Virginia, routinely talks to his unconscious patients as he finishes the operation. To a patient having a hip replacement, he says, "I am pleased with your new hip." Several patients have told him that his words reassured them. He is also Associate Clinical Professor of Orthopedics at the University of Virginia Health Sciences.

Cancer

I have been asked, "What if the doctor discovered cancer?" In this situation, it is even more important to hear the positive statement that you are doing fine when you are highly suggestible. Finding cancer is not a death sentence. It means cancer was found and you have great healing capacities that need to be mobilized.

For example, a research study showed when patients with breast cancer used relaxation and visualization to reduce stress there was an increase in immune function as measured by natural killer (NK) cell cytotoxicity and IL-2-activated NK cell activity. This study was done at the University of South Florida College of Nursing. Findings were published in *Biological Research for Nursing* in 2008.[15-18]

What Has Suppressed Your Immune System?

When cancer is involved, it is time to ask a question: What ongoing stresses during the past few years have been suppressing my immune system?

When I've asked clients, I often hear, "Oh, the last three years were awful. My father had open-heart surgery and I had a boss who never got off my case. At work my stomach was always tied in knots."

If you have been chronically tense, this will have caused your sympathetic nervous system to be dominant. While it gave you surges of stress hormones such as adrenaline to get through crisis after crisis, it suppressed your immune system, leaving you susceptible to illness.

You can restore your immune system by taking the necessary steps to create peace where there was anxiety. The epilogue shows you how to reduce stress and feel peaceful.

In addition, take the vitamins, exercise and diet that boost your immune system. Along with the treatment plan recommended by your doctors, a strengthened immune system is a major factor that contributes to the remission of cancer.

For an inspiring book which will guide and empower you, read *Crazy Sexy Cancer Tips* by Kris Carr.

Third Healing Statement:

"Following this operation, you will be hungry for _____. You will be thirsty and urinate easily."

Fill in the blank with your favorite drink or light food, such as tea, apple juice or chicken soup.

This statement tells your digestive and elimination systems to wake up and start working again. It helps avoid the medical complications that can arise when these systems are sluggish from anesthesia.

The suggestion of your favorite light food stimulates your appetite, so that you are likely to be hungry after the operation. Tea or chicken soup are easy for your stomach to digest after surgery.

The benefits of waking up the elimination system were documented in a study at the University of California, Davis Medical Center. Patients given therapeutic suggestions moved their bowels in an average of 2.6 days, as compared to 4.2 days for the patients in the control group. They left the hospital 1.5 days sooner, at a savings of about $1,200 per person.[19]

The study was conducted by Elizabeth Disbrow and Dr. Henry L. Bennett, an Associate Professor in the Department of Anesthesiology. He has done pioneering work, documenting the effects of positive suggestion during surgery.

When Not Allowed to Drink Liquid after Surgery
If your type of surgery does not allow you to drink liquid after surgery, change the Third Healiung Statement. Use only "Following this operation, you will urinate easily". Cross out the first sentence, "Following this operation you will be hungry for_____".

For example, bariatric surgery for weight loss and other gastrointestinal surgeries require that you not drink or eat anything after surgery until a test shows your gastrointestinal tract is functioning.

Fourth Healing Statement: *(optional)*

"Following this operation, _____."

It is optional to use the Fourth Healing Statement.

If you use it, fill in the blank with the words your surgeon recommends for your recovery. The sentence should be extremely positive, clearly spelling out the specific suggestions that will speed your recovery.

Ask your doctor to describe your healing process in words and pictures, explaining the physiology of your recovery. With this specific information, you and your doctor can draft the statement.

If you have already met with your surgeon, you can obtain this information by phone. Ask the surgeon's secretary to arrange a telephone meeting with your doctor or one of the residents.

Four months after a mastectomy, Joan Irving, an actress in New York City, was preparing for reconstructive surgery of her right breast. Her surgeon, Dr. Randolph Guthrie, explained that the skin on her right chest had to stretch to accommodate the implant.

Understanding the physical details of her recovery, Joan wrote, "Following this operation the skin on your chest will comfortably stretch to accommodate the implant in your right chest."

Dr. Guthrie repeated this statement five times towards the end of Joan's surgery. During her recuperation, Joan's chest felt comfortable, instead of the tight, stretching sensation often experienced.

The benefits of using therapeutic statements about recovery have been well documented in a study by Dr. Willard Mainord, a psychologist in Kentucky. To facilitate patients' healing from back surgery,

Dr. Mainord had the surgeon say the following words to the patient during surgery:

> You will be flat on your back for the next couple of days. While you are waiting, it would be a good idea if you relax the muscles in the pelvic area, as this will enable you to urinate and it will not be necessary to use a catheter.

The 12 people who heard these words had the same operation with the same surgeon. Following surgery, all 12 avoided needing a catheter to urinate. However, in the control group, five of the 12 people required a catheter.

According to Dr. Mainord, "This is a success rate that has only a 3 in 1,000 chance of occurring."[20]

To corroborate his findings, Dr. Mainord asked neuropsychologist Dr. Barry Rath to do a similar study. Using 44 people, Dr. Rath gave half the anesthetized patients the following suggestion during surgery, "You will feel little pain. You will be able to urinate easily and you will recover quickly." To the control group, he said a "nonsense" message, "It's a beautiful day."

The results were similar to Dr. Mainord's. Patients hearing the positive statements reported less pain, used less pain medication and left the hospital 1.5 days earlier than the control group.[21]

When to Call Dept. of Anesthesia

A few days before surgery, call the Dept. of Anesthesia to be sure you will have an anesthesiologist or nurse in the operating room who will be glad to say the Healing Statements. You only need to do this if it is not routine practice for your hopsital to use Healing Statements.

If you do not have a preoperative meeting, *preops*, you will need to call the Dept. of Anesthesia to request that an anesthesiologist or nurse in the operating room is assigned to your case to say the Healing Statements.

Three Pages of the Healing Statements

Three pages of the Healing Statements are on pages 259–263. Cut them out of the book. This leaves a permanent copy of the statements on page 171, in case you loan the book to a friend who is facing surgery.

* **Give one page to your surgeon.**
* **Second page is for an anesthesiologist at *preops*.**
* **Bring the third to the hospital on the day of surgery to give to your anesthesiologist.**

Scotch-tape the third page to your hospital gown so it is visible. Don't use a safety pin. It's not safe and will only be removed.

When your anesthesiologist meets you 30 minutes before surgery, ask him or her to say the Healing Statements during surgery. *As a patient, it is your legal right to request them and have them used.*

Block Out Operating Room Conversations

Whether you will be conscious or unconscious, it is important to protect yourself from hearing operating room conversations that you might interpret negatively. Block them out by listening to the Relaxation CD once the First Healing Statement has been repeated five times at the beginning of surgery.

If you will be awake during surgery, you may prefer not to hear the doctors and nurses talking over your body. Even if your operation is a standard procedure, it's often a shock to hear them casually discussing basketball scores or their weekend plans while they tie your sutures.

Operating Room Noise

The level of noise in an operating room has been documented by Marcia Steinberg, CNOR, a nurse anesthetist at Emory University School of Medicine in Atlanta. During her own surgery, she found that a preoperative dose of Demerol heightened her sense of hearing, magnifying all the sounds in the operating room. She was alarmed by the level of noise and concerned about how other patients might be affected by it.

In the operating room, doctors and nurses talk, machines bleep, steel surgical instruments clank as they are dropped into metal pans and music plays over the loudspeakers.

In a New York City hospital, one surgeon, an amateur drummer, has even been known to beat time to Frank Sinatra on the patient's metal retractors, the clamps that hold the incision open.

All those sounds bouncing off tile walls create a considerable din. Using acoustical equipment to measure operating room noise, Marcia Steinberg, CNOR, documented bursts of sound equal to a jet during take-off.

Healing Power of Music

Protect yourself from the noise by listening to the Relaxation CD during surgery. If you have an iPod, transfer the Relaxation CD to it. If you'd like, add music, alternating 20 minutes of the Relaxation CD with your favorite music. If you need help, ask a friend who uses an iPod to show you how to do this.

Whether it is Bach, Beethoven or the Beatles, all music affects your emotions. Certain songs soothe. Others inspire exalted feelings. Some make you lonely and depressed.

Select music that you love that lifts your spirit. It will help your healing.

When you tap your foot to music, you feel its tempo. In the Renaissance, the tempo of music was the normal heart rate, 70 to 80 beats a minute. When you listen to faster music, its beat speeds up your heart rate. Therefore, select classical or popular music that is calming. Research indicates it will slow your heart beat and lower your blood pressure.[22-26]

Music Reduces Pain and Anxiety
Studies also reveal that quieting music reduces anxiety and lessens the need for pain medication. It is thought that soothing music helps produce the peptides in the brain that relieve pain.

While many studies have documented the healing benefits of music, one of the most interesting was conducted by music therapist Dr. Helen Bonney in the coronary-care units of two hospitals, St. Agnes Hospital in Baltimore, Maryland, and Jefferson General Hospital in Port Townsend, Washington. When soothing music was played, patients needed less medication for pain and anxiety.[27]

Auto-Play CD Player or iPod
Use an auto-play CD or iPod so that the Relaxation CD and music will play throughout the operation. At home, make sure it is in working order. Test the earphones and set the volume at a comfortable level. Put scotch-tape on the volume control to keep it from being moved.

Turn the auto-play on and tape all the controls so they cannot be accidentally turned off. The day before you go to the hospital, insert new batteries in your player. Take the electric cord to the hospital in case you need to recharge your iPod.

Permission to Use CD or iPod

Ask if you will need permission to bring your CD player or iPod in the operating room. Some hospitals require permission. Make this arrangement during your preoperative meeting at the hospital or call PreAdmissions to ask someone to get permission.

You can also arrange permission to keep religious medals, wigs or dentures near you with your medical chart during surgery. Some people are more comfortable putting on their wig or popping in their dentures as soon as they regain consciousness.

Hospitals want you to be comfortable. As a result, these arrangements are easy to make. Write down the name of the person who gave you permission, in case you get to the hospital and it has not been written on your medical chart.

Ear Plugs Don't Block Out All Sounds

If you are thinking of using ear plugs to block out the operating room conversations, don't. Ear plugs block out some of the sounds but you can still hear.

Protect Yourself from Hearing Diagnosis

As a child on your way home from school, did you ever write your name in wet cement? If so, remember how your writing hardened into concrete. This is how your doctor's diagnosis will be imprinted on your unconscious mind if you cannot block it out.

Whether you will be unconscious or conscious, you will be in a deep altered state of consciousness in which few of your mental filters, which normally process information in a waking state, will be functioning. As a result, you are like a blank slate that can be written upon, without the ability to accept or reject the doctor's prognosis for your life.

Even when you are fully conscious its a major task not to be negatively influenced by your doctor's evaluation of your condition.

If there is any possibility that you might have a serious diagnosis during surgery, such as a biopsy revealing cancer, it is very important that you do not hear this information during the operation when you are highly suggestible.

When you are awake and fully conscious, it is a much better time to hear your diagnosis. If you find that you have cancer, you will be able to ask your doctor about all of the options for treatment.

Tell your surgeon that you want to be given this information when you have fully regained consciousness and not in the recovery room.

Your request prevents your surgeon from telling you a negative prognosis while you are still drowsy from the anesthesia and <u>highly suggestible</u>.

Roused from Semi-Consciousness

Marjie Thorne, of Concord, Massachusetts, vividly remembers her doctor rousing her from semi-consciousness in the recovery room to tell her the results of her breast biopsy. While her surgeon thought he was doing the best thing, she remembers the effect. Hearing the diagnosis of cancer, she sank into a deep depression.

Marjie was very depressed for several weeks until friends urged her to rally and seek second opinions from other doctors.

Marjie's reaction to her diagnosis was fortunately counterbalanced by her meeting with Dr. Susan Troyan at one of the Harvard Medical School teaching hospitals.

Hope

Marjie had gone to Dr. Troyan for a second opinion about her treatment. On a Friday afternoon of a hot summer day Dr. Troyan talked to Marjie, putting her X-rays on a light box so that Marjie could understand them.

When Dr. Troyan took the time to explain how the tumor might have developed and how, with treatment, her outcome was optimistic, Marjie's hope was restored. In turn, Marjie's hope dispelled her depression the way the sun burns off an early morning fog.

Hope and optimism are important attitudes. Many studies indicate that optimistic people are healthier and outlive their pessimistic counterparts.

If you're a pessimist, this is an attitude you can change. Dr. Aaron Beck, a psychiatrist at the University of Pennsylvania, explains how in a book, *Feeling Good.* Also read *Positivity*, by Barbara L. Fredrickson, Ph.D., a leader in the field of positive psychology.

Pathologist's Report

Unfortunately for patients, many hospitals have the pathologist's report announced over a loudspeaker in the operating room. While it lets the surgeon hear the report while operating, patients also hear it whether they are conscious or unconscious.

In other hospitals, the surgeon walks a few steps to a telephone where the pathologist gives the report in private.

Listening to music will protect you from hearing the report or your surgeon discussing it with other doctors in the operating room.

While scientists are still trying to understand the mechanisms of consciousness that allow so-called unconscious patients to hear, it is important to remember how highly suggestible you are during surgery, whether you are awake or unconscious.

What your doctors say can either greatly help or hinder your recovery. [28-31]

Three pages of Healing Statements are at the back of the book beginning on page 259. If you need to use them, cut them out.

Leave page 171 as a permanent page of Healing Statements in the book.

Peggy Huddleston's
Healing Statements for Surgery

Patient's Name _____

(Give this page to your surgeon and another to your anesthesiologist. Tape a third page to your hospital gown, so it is visible as you go into surgery.)

As I am going under the anesthesia, please say:

1. "Following this operation, you will feel comfortable and you will heal very well." (Repeat 5 times.)

After saying the statements, please put on my earphones and start my CD or iPod.

Towards the end of surgery, remove my earphones. Say:

2. "Your operation has gone very well." (Repeat 5 times.)

3. "Following this operation, you will be hungry for _____. You will be thirsty and urinate easily." (Repeat 5 times.)

4. "Following this operation _____
_____."
Fill in your surgeon's recommendations for recovery. (Repeat 5 times.)

I am allergic to these anesthesias and medications:

The medications and the dosages I am taking are:

© Peggy Huddleston, *Prepare for Surgery, Heal Faster: A Guide of Mind-Body Techniques* (Cambridge, MA; Angel River Press; Fourth Edition, 2012).

Summary

Step 4
Use Healing Statements

1. After all your questions are answered, explain to your surgeon, "There are some Healing Statements that I would like you or the anesthesiologist to say to me during my operation. The first is said as I go under to anesthesia. The others are said towards the end of the operation."

2. If you will be awake during surgery, explain that the first Healing Statement is said as you are deeply relaxed at the beginning of surgery.

3. Give your surgeon a page of the Healing Statements on page 259, having filled in the blanks.

4. With your surgeon, decide who is the best person to read them, your surgeon, the anesthesiologist or a nurse in the operating room.

5. Even if the anesthesiologist will say them, explain them to your surgeon so that he or she can be supportive of their use.

6. The first statement, to be repeated five times, is, "Following this operation, you will feel comfortable and you will heal very well."

7. After it has been spoken, ask that your CD or iPod be turned on and the earphones put in your ears to protect you from hearing operating room noise and conversations.

8. Explain that the other Healing Statements are to be said five times towards the end of surgery, after removing your earphones.

"Your operation has gone very well."
(Fill in the blank.) Repeat five times.

"Following this operation, you will be hungry for _____. You will be thirsty and urinate easily."

(Fill in the blank.) Repeat five times.

9. If you will be awake during surgery, having local or regional anesthesia, tell your surgeon, "After the first Healing Statement and during the operation, I will be listening to a CD or iPod as a way to relax.

10. If you are using a CD player or iPod during your operation, set the volume. Put scotch-tape on the controls so that they can't be accidentally changed. Insert new batteries. Be sure it works.

11. Ask your surgeon when will you have your preoperative meeting and talk to an anesthesiologist.

12. On the day of surgery, scotch-tape the page of Healing Statements to your hospital gown. Your anesthesiologist will see them when he or she meets you before surgery.

13. Ask if you'll need patient-controlled analgesia (PCA) following surgery.

14. Add your ideas here:

Peggy Huddleston's
Healing Statements for Surgery

Patient's Name _____

(Give this page to your surgeon and another to your anesthesiologist. Tape a third page to your hospital gown, so it is visible as you go into surgery.)

As I am going under the anesthesia, please say:

1. "Following this operation, you will feel comfortable and you will heal very well." (Repeat 5 times.)

After saying the statements, please put on my earphones and start my CD or iPod.

Towards the end of surgery, remove my earphones. Say:

2. "Your operation has gone very well." (Repeat 5 times.)

3. "Following this operation, you will be hungry for _____. You will be thirsty and urinate easily." (Repeat 5 times.)

4. "Following this operation _____
_____."
Fill in your surgeon's recommendations for recovery. (Repeat 5 times.)

I am allergic to these anesthesias and medications:

The medications and the dosages I am taking are:

© Peggy Huddleston, *Prepare for Surgery, Heal Faster: A Guide of Mind-Body Techniques* (Cambridge, MA; Angel River Press; Fourth Edition, 2012).

Step 5

Meet
An Anesthesiologist

He visits patients the night before an
operation and, if he gains rapport, confidence
and trust, knows that he will give less an
aesthetic the next day.
— J.N. Blau

For years anesthesiologists have combined drugs to
calm patients before surgery. It turns out that one of
the most active ingredients for calming you is
not a drug, but rather an informative and
supportive doctor-patient relationship with an
anesthesiologist. It puts your mind at ease to have
your questions answered and meet the doctor to
whom you'll entrust yourself.

The value of meeting your anesthesiologist prior to
surgery has been well documented. In a study at the

Anaesthesia Laboratory of Harvard Medical School at Massachusetts General Hospital, Dr. Lawrence Egbert worked with 218 patients awaiting surgery. At random, they were given a dose of the sedative Pentobarbital or a five-to 10-minute reassuring meeting with an anesthesiologist.

The results showed that meeting the doctor had a much more calming effect than the drug. The patients who received the drug felt drowsy, but still nervous. In comparison, the patients who met the anesthesiologists reported feeling calm before surgery.[1]

Dr. Egbert conducted another study in which the anesthesiologists had supportive meetings with their patients, 97 adults about to undergo elective intra-abdominal operations. In addition, 46 of those patients were instructed in how to reduce their postoperative pain by relaxing their abdominal muscles. Specifically, the patients were shown how to turn over in bed, using their arms and legs while relaxing their abdominal muscles.

Dr. Egbert reported in *The New England Journal of Medicine*: "In the afternoon after the operation, the anesthetists again visited their 46 patients. The doctors reiterated what they had taught the patients the night before and reassured them that the discomfort or pain that they were experiencing was normal. All this was repeated once or twice a day until the patients had no further need of narcotics."

Ultimately, the patients receiving the special instructions used 50% less pain medication and went home 2.7 days earlier than the control group.[2]

Dr. Egbert's research shows how important it is to meet your anesthesiologist before surgery. However, in most hospitals in America, your anesthesiologist is not assigned to your case until the day before surgery or even the morning of surgery which makes it difficult to meet this doctor.

Fortunately, you do meet with an anesthesiologist at your preoperative meeting, called *preops*, which is a week or a few days before surgery. This is the time to get your questions answered and ask that an anesthesiologist be assigned to you who will be glad to say the Healing Statements. Hospitals are glad to do this.

Make a List of Questions about the Anesthesia
Decide in advance how much medical information you want to hear. The anesthesiologist will be guided by your questions and will be glad to provide the information you want. It's up to you to express your needs clearly.

Will you need preoperative medication? If so, make sure it matches your coping style. Tell the doctor if you plan to listen to the Relaxation CD to calm yourself before surgery.

You may not need any preoperative medication, but if you do, it should work with your natural coping style. The wrong preoperative medication can actually create stress.

For example, people whose coping style is vigilant like being in control and knowing lots of medical details about their surgery. They rely on their minds and thinking as a way of feeling safe. If people with that coping style are given scopolamine, a drug that depletes certain brain neurotransmitters making it hard to hang on to thoughts, they may become quite stressed.

In some cases, Valium® (diazepam) or morphine would be more appropriate because they relax the body like a rag doll, while allowing the mind to go on thinking. These medications would let your mind function enough to listen to the Relaxation CD.

The opposite coping style is avoiding and denying. People who cope this way feel better pulling the covers over their head and going to sleep when confronted with a problem. They cope by blocking out the problem, denying that it even exists. Those people prefer having a drug that simply blanks out their mind and drains away their attention, so they can't think.

If this is your coping style, and you are not having preoperative medication, use the Relaxation CD as a way to disassociate from the preoperative situation. Having the CD guide you through a process of deep relaxation in which you imagine your favorite beach will distract you from the hospital noise and any preoperative procedures.

Whatever your coping style, it's not likely to change. It is important that you know yourself and alert your doctors so they can cooperate with your style of coping, rather than unknowingly working against it. With the right medication or even no medication, you can feel peaceful before surgery.

If you will be awake during surgery, ask the doctor to explain the procedure for the local or regional anesthesia.
What should you expect to feel? You'll feel better prepared knowing what to expect. If you plan to listen to the Relaxation CD during surgery, tell your doctor.

If you will be unconscious during surgery, discuss what the anesthesiologist will say to you as you go under the anesthesia.
As you are given the anesthesia, some anesthesiologists like to use imagery, saying, "Imagine yourself on a beautiful beach." If you hate beaches, that's the last thing you want to hear.

Choose a scene that is right for you. Tell the anesthesiologist the scene so that he or she can tell your actual anesthesiologist to evoke this image. One woman asked her doctor to say, "Imagine yourself being held in the arms of your husband." Those words made her feel safe as the anesthesia took effect.

Some people have memories of being tricked as children when they were given anesthesia before their tonsils or appendix were taken out. Without any explanation that they were about to become unconscious, their doctor said, "Just blow into this red balloon."

If you were tricked like this as a child, tell your anesthesiologist. As an adult, you'll have an opportunity to rework this event with a doctor who can create a trusting experience.

Explain how you would like to be treated as you are given the anesthesia.

You may want your anesthesiologist to hold your hand or stroke your forehead as you go under the anesthesia. Dr. Susan M. Love, surgeon and author of *Dr. Susan Love's Breast Book,* likes to hold a patient's hand and talk as the patient goes under the anesthesia.

If you have any fears about the anesthesia, talk these over with your doctor.

Your anesthesiologist can tell you various ways of solving those concerns. Usually your fears can be allayed with straightforward information about what will happen. If you've had bad experiences during an earlier surgery, tell your doctor, so that he or she can avoid a reoccurrence.

If you ever had awareness during a previous surgery, you will be relieved to know there is a way to avoid it. Tell the anesthesiologist about your experience and request that a BIS Monitor be used when you have surgery. It monitors the depth of anesthesia so the anesthesiologist is sure you have adequate amounts of anesthesia.

Request Use of Healing Statements.

Tell the anesthesiologist you are using this book and a Relaxation CD to prepare for surgery. Ask to have an anesthesiologist assigned to your case who will be glad to say the Healing Statements. Give the doctor the page of Healing Statements which you have cut out of the book.

Even if your surgeon delivers the statements, your anesthesiologist should still be aware and supportive of them. Also invite your anesthesiologist to express any spontaneous, positive statements during the operation.

Discuss Your Medications and Allergies.

On the page of Healing Statements, write the names of all the medications you are taking. Also list the names of any drugs or anesthesias to which you are allergic. Carefully review this information with the anesthesiologist, asking if there are any medications you should stop taking before surgery.

This helps avoid the risk of harmful drug interactions. Even though your doctors will ask about allergic reactions, you should also be responsible for communicating that information.

If you take tranquilizers, tell your doctor what your usual dose is. If you drink wine or alcohol, tell your doctor how much is too much. Those guidelines will help the anesthesiologist evaluate your responsiveness to sedatives and narcotics. If you use marijuana or take drugs, tell this doctor.

If you are a member of Alcoholics Anonymous or have had a drinking problem, be sure to say so and write it on the page. The information will help your doctor evaluate your tolerance for chemicals. Even if you have been sober for many years, your sensitivity to chemicals may mean you'll require less anesthesia.

If you are a member of Overeaters Anonymous or avoid any form of sugar, ask to be given a saline solution instead of an intravenous fluid containing dextrose. The saline solution is not a food source but should suffice for a short amount of time. Also ask your anesthesiologist about other sources of nutrition.

When should you stop eating or drinking the night before surgery?

The cut off times for food and liquids are crucial. If you ingest anything after this time, the operation will have to be canceled.

Eating and drinking nothing, not even a sip of water, could save your life. If you have water or food in your stomach during surgery, you run the risk of aspirating. This means you vomit. Because you are likely to be lying on your back in the operating room, the contents of your stomach could go into your windpipe and lungs, blocking your breathing, creating a life-threatening situation.

ₗne best way to prevent this is to follow the doctor's rules. If you have eaten something, tell your surgeon so that your surgery can be delayed until your stomach is completely empty. In the hospital, if you see a sign on your door saying: NPO. That's Latin for nil per os, meaning nothing by mouth.

What medications will be available to reduce postoperative discomfort or pain?

Will you have patient-control analgesia (PCA) and be able to give yourself pain medication? If not, find out how to get pain medication if you need it. The more you know about the hospital's procedures, the more in control you will be after your operation.

Your Surgeon's Instructions

Your surgeon will tell you what to expect after surgery and how to take care of yourself during your recovery. Find out if you will have any drainage tubes and how they will affect your ability to turn over or cough. If you are having abdominal surgery, learn the trick of holding a pillow against your stomach muscles, making coughing or laughing bearable.

As you can see, an informative and supportive meeting goes a long way toward reducing your stress and preparing you for an optimal outcome.

In Recovery Room Listen to CD

In the recovery room, listening to the Relaxation CD reduces discomfort and helps you feel peaceful. You will be thirsty for your favorite drink or light food which will wake up your digestive tract and help your vital signs get back to normal much sooner.

You can have your favorite drink or light food as soon as you get home if you are having day surgery or as soon as you get to your hospital room if you are spending the night there.

Nurses in the recovery room at Brigham and Women's Hospital in Boston say that patients using this book and Relaxation CD wake up from the anesthesia smiling and have their vital signs return to normal one to three hours sooner than patients not using them.

Change Your First End-Result

Once your first end-result has happened change it to be your goal for your recovery for each day. If you are in the hospital, ask your nurse, "What are your goals for me today?" Your nurse may say, "I want to get you out of bed and have you walk to the end of the hall and back to your bed."

Listen to the Relaxation CD, feeling like you already have **triumphantly** walked to the end of the hall and back to your bed.

Everyday, ask your nurse, "What are your goals for me today?" and again make them your first end-result.

Listen to CD beforePhysical Therapy

If you are having physical therapy before or after surgery, you will have less discomfort and more range of motion if you listen to the Relaxation CD 30 minutes before it. The relaxation soothes your muscles and tendons which makes physical therapy easier. Many orthopedic surgeons have been surprised and pleased by the excellent range of motion their patients achieved using *Prepare for Surgery, Heal Faster.*

Research Study with Knee-Joint Replacement

A randomized, controlled study with 44 patients having total knee-joint replacement documented that patients using this book and Relaxation tape and a one-hour *Prepare for Surgery, Heal Faster Workshop* had significantly less anxiety the day before surgery. They were discharged from the hospital 1.3 days sooner than those in the control group.

This study was done with Benjamin E. Bierbaum, MD, the former Chief of Orthopedic Surgery at the New England Baptist Hospital, a Tufts University School of Medicine teaching hospital.[3] Abstract on page 249.

Discharged from the Hospital
When you are discharged from the hospital, you will be given written instructions about how to change the dressing on your surgical wound and how to limit your physical activity while you are healing.

Even if you are healing faster than expected, follow your surgeon's written guidelines for resuming physical activities.

Many people who used this method to prepare for surgery asked me to tell you not to over do physical activities during your recovery just because you feel fine. Enjoy feeling well and take it easy.

Congratulations!
You have come to the end of the five steps. By putting them into practice, you will have done a lot to prepare for surgery. You can easily stop here.

But some people have the desire to do more. If you do, read on. The epilogue shows you an additional way to enhance your healing, using inner peace and love.

As you read the epilogue, you'll know if it is for you. It could be just what you are looking for now. If not, you may want to use it in the future.

Summary

Step 5
Meet An Anesthesiologist

1. You will meet with an anesthesiologist a few days or a week before surgery during your preoperative meeting.

2. Make a list of questions you want to ask about the anesthesia and the procedure.

3. If you need preoperative medication, inquire if it matches your coping style.

4. If you will be awake during your operation, ask the doctor to explain the procedure for the local or regional anesthesia.

5. If you will be unconscious during surgery, discuss what will be said to you as you are given the anesthesia. Choose a scene to visualize that is safe and comforting.

6. Tell this anesthesiologist how you would like to be treated as you are given the anesthesia. Would you like your hand held or forehead stroked? If you have worries about the anesthesia, talk them over.

7. At the preoperative meeting, give the anesthesi-ologist the page of Healing Statements. Even if your surgeon is the one to say them, go over them with this anesthesiologist.

8. To avoid harmful drug interactions, write the names of all the medications you are taking on the page of Healing Statements. List the names of drugs or anesthesias to which you are allergic.

9. Find out the exact time you should stop eating or drinking the night before your operation. Surgery needs to be delayed until your stomach is empty.

10. What medications will be available for you to reduce any postoperative discomfort or pain? Will you have patient-controlled analgesia (PCA)?

11. Ask for specific instructions about how to move and care for your body after surgery.

12. Add your ideas here:

Epilogue

One More Way
to Enhance Healing

> ...when you feel as your only need that
> need to travel deeper into your own soul...

> — Karen Goldman

Deep within you, perhaps forgotten or buried long ago, is a place of immense peace. It is a source of ever flowing love. It is your essence.

You can block your experience of this love or learn to access it with enormous benefit to your life. In the epilogue, you'll discover ways of opening to this peace. It will enhance the healing of your body, mind and soul.

When Christina Walters of Dublin, New Hampshire, called me about preparing for surgery, I asked her, "When do you feel a sense of oneness or an inner peace?" She answered, "Sitting on my porch, watching the hummingbirds at the feeder. As I gaze at them, I become one with the trees and sky. I feel such a peace."

I asked how often she did that, "Oh, only for five minutes in the morning," she replied. "I always feel I should go in the house and do something useful, like make the beds."

I explained that before and after surgery, one of the most useful things she could do was watch the hummingbirds. By letting the serenity of the scene flow through her for as long as she liked, she would be calm during the two weeks before surgery. The tranquility would strengthen her immune system. After her operation, she could use the peace to facilitate her healing.

Prescription
As a prescription, I asked her to watch the hummingbirds for at least 15 minutes, three times a day. She took a deep breath and said, "How wonderful to do that, knowing it's constructive."

She chose the 15 minutes after breakfast, lunch and dinner. It is best to be specific about the times and even write them in your calendar to save the time for yourself. It is an important meeting with peace. If something comes up and you cancel the meeting, be sure to reschedule it.

After a week of absorbing the serenity, Christine extended each of the 15 minutes to half an hour. She was comfortable being immersed in the peace for longer stretches of time. Whenever she was overwhelmed by fears about the operation, she imagined the hummingbirds and a sense of presence would come over her.

With her new skill of calling up the peace at will, she could shift herself out of her anxiety, stopping the flight-or-fight response. Preparing for surgery in this way allowed her to relax, using all of her energy to strengthen her immune system.

After surgery, when she felt any discomfort or pain, imagining the hummingbirds and feeling the peace diminished it. As the tranquility soothed her — physically, emotionally and spiritually — she knew this way of "being" was profoundly healing.

Find the Doorways to Oneness

While the hummingbirds were Christina's way of experiencing oneness, Joe Trujillo, a staff member of the United States Senate in Washington, D.C., uses music as the key to open the door to the transpersonal dimension. Whenever he hears Eric Clapton and Cream singing "Crossroads" and "Spoonful," Joe is uplifted and filled with oneness.

For Juliette Montague, a lawyer in Boston, Massachusetts, visiting Vermont connects her with an inner peace. The barns, trees and the countryside — everything she sees, transports her into a sense of oneness. She loves how the land rolls and peaks, as the back roads follow the river valleys. She says, "Driving down a country road, I feel as if I'm not in the car but flying through the land."

For Fredrica Wagman, a novelist in Philadelphia, writing pushes open the door to this dimension. She says, "When I'm writing, I'm in the arms of God, being kissed — surrounded by love."

As a child, Tricia Bracken, a court stenographer in Taunton, Massachusetts, remembers always feeling euphoric — until she was 14. She says, "Our house was filled with lots of cousins, running and playing. As a child, I loved to play, but gradually, that feeling of oneness slipped away as I went to work and had to be responsible. Since then I think about that feeling all the time, and I'm waiting for it to come back."

All of these individuals were getting in touch with an aspect of their being that helped them feel peaceful, more complete — whole.

When "Something is Missing"

When people feel that "something is missing" in their lives, often what is missing is their connection to this dimension. Dr. Carl G. Jung, the Swiss psychiatrist, referred to this loss of connection to something larger than themselves as the cause of alienation in modern Western society.

When people feel alienated and alone, they are disconnected from this ground of being — this energy which literally nurtures your soul.

When we do not feel whole, we search for something outside of ourselves to complete us, such as the right job or the right relationship. Most advertising is based on this primal, unconscious need, offering us products to fill the empty place inside.

But they can never fill it. Instead, we need to open to the oneness that is within us, around us and is us. It gives us a sense of wholeness — a sense of coming home.

Web of Life

Many indigenous peoples, such as the aborigines of Australia or the Native American tribes, the Lakota and the Cherokee, are deeply rooted in oneness. Their ancient traditions taught that they were one with everything — the earth, trees, stars and the cosmos. Lakota children could easily merge their beings with an eagle, soaring with it through the clouds.

Many of their rituals reinforced their sense of the interconnectedness of life. They call it the "web of life." Sadly, in many parts of the world those traditions have been eroded by the influences of Western civilization that is blind to the web of life that connects us all in oneness.

In preparing for and recovering from surgery or any illness, you'll want to find the keys that open the doors to this transpersonal dimension. By dwelling in it, you'll facilitate your healing process on all levels of your body, mind and soul.

Unfortunately, our Western society does not teach us as children how to connect with the transpersonal dimension. But it is always there. Maybe you have already discovered it. Perhaps as a young child you lay in the tall grass watching the swallows and found that you could swoop with them.

Maybe you played in the woods, and as you become one with the squirrels and the blue jays, you discovered that inner peace. Or perhaps you were like Tricia Bracken and experienced a sense of euphoria in your everyday childhood world.

Doing What You Love
Doing the things that you love will often open you up to the transpersonal dimension. Absorbed in the "doing," you experience your own "being."

For example, when you see "a star at dawn, a bubble in a stream or a flash of lightning in a summer cloud" you feel moved. It is your being, your essence, that is touched. Opening up to your own being, letting it be moved by beauty, is deeply healing.

You are removing the blocks to your being. You are coming face to face with your essence.

Being Versus Doing

Unfortunately, our society does not reward "being." Instead, it values doing — closing one more deal, writing one more report and completing one more project.

To achieve more, you think faster, juggling two or three things at a time. We even install telephones in our bathrooms, pockets and cars so we can get more done. Modern life becomes a compulsive blur of deadlines and goals.

The myth of success leads to what mythologist Joseph Campbell called "climbing the ladder only to discover it was against the wrong wall."

On our deathbeds, we don't remember our worldly accomplishments. If we recall anything, we recall the times we loved, as memories of them involuntarily flash in front of our eyes. They are our true accomplishments.

Learning the art of "being" is quite different from doing. Instead of racing into the future, you'll find yourself slowing down, living in the moment as you watch the sun rise or the wonder of a child sleeping.

You experience the transpersonal dimension through your feelings rather than your mind. You feel the beauty of the sunlight glistening on the water. You feel uplifted by the sweeping music. You feel the joy of being with someone you love.

You'll notice that as your capacity to feel increases your mind becomes quieter — until it is still. It's an awakening to the moment.

Open Your Capacity to Feel

If you have numbed your capacity to feel as a way to avoid your emotions, learning to relax is a gentle way to open up feeling. Colors become brighter, food tastes better and you feel more alive.

Paradoxically, you experience inner peace or oneness by letting go, rather than grasping it. If you remember times when you felt a sense of oneness, it just happened.

To cultivate being, make a list of the things that nurture you. Yours might include: having a massage, soaking in a hot bath surrounded by candlelight and music, making love, arranging flowers, baking bread, painting, listening to music or watching clouds drift across the sky.

You can experience all of these, the massage or the bath, in an ordinary state of mind, where your mind is always the observer, where there is a subject and an object. Or you can shift into being by becoming absorbed with the experience.

Many experience this fusion with oneness as their natural state. Indeed, it should be.

Do the things that you love just for the pure joy of it. If you do any as a task, you'll be defeating the purpose. It's being a child again. Playing for the fun of it. Remember how you jumped in puddles, climbed trees, blew bubbles and had pillow fights.

The transpersonal dimension is the same as the ecstatic world of a happy child. To join the grown-up world, the child has to pull back from the sheer joy of life.

In the words of the French poet Stéphane Mallarmé: The child abdicates his ecstasy ("L'enfant abdique son extase."). Now you are reversing that process.

Your Capacity for Joy

Your capacity for joy was shaped by the family in which you grew up. From them, you may have learned to put a ceiling on how happy you can be. While you are healing, you want to push through this ceiling.

You can easily expand beyond any limits set by your family.

Nancy Versis remembers as a child exuberantly splashing in a sink full of water. As she laughed with delight, she could feel that her expansive joy made her mother cringe. In that moment, she decided it was not safe to feel so much joy. Growing up, she always kept a lid on getting too happy so that her mother would not pull away.

Cultural Beliefs

Similarly, the values and beliefs of the culture you grew up in also influence how acceptable it is to experience joy. For example, when I moved from Philadelphia to Cambridge, Massachusetts, for graduate study at Harvard Divinity School, I was taken aback by my New England friends' reaction to a hot chocolate souffle I had made for dessert.

As they ate the souffle, they said, "It's so good, it's sinful." In modern Puritan New England, something could still be so good it was sinful.

In my psychotherapy practice in Cambridge, I discovered that several people often had migraine headaches during their vacations in Bermuda or Maine. Their Yankee upbringing had filled them with the belief that it was virtuous only to work hard and be industrious. Taking a vacation was not acceptable.

In the early Puritan days, a frontier society pushing back the wilderness had made hard work the dominant virtue. There was no place for pleasure, except to call it "sinful" or "the work of the devil."

Three hundred years later those unexamined beliefs were causing migraine headaches in a New Englander lying on the pink sand beaches of Bermuda.

Examine Your Limiting Beliefs

If you are from a Puritan, Calvinist or a similarly austere background that limits pleasure, you'll need to examine your own beliefs, changing them to make room for more joy.

Likewise, if you are from a tradition in which suffering is a virtue and pleasure is considered bad, you'll have to work your way through altering those beliefs. In those traditions, hardship and abuse were endured because of the belief that if something hurt, it must be good.

This in turn created the idea that if something felt good, it must be wrong. By changing those beliefs, you'll give yourself permission to experience more joy.

Your Need for Nurturing

If the thought of feeling happier stirs up an inner voice saying, "You'll become lazy or selfish," discover what family or cultural voice is speaking. If you are afraid of indulging yourself too much, becoming narcissistic, be assured that you need to give in to the part of you that feels deprived. You probably never got the nurturing you needed as a child.

In addition, you may even have learned to feel ashamed of your needs for love and recognition. Narcissism is the opposite of what it looks like. Narcissists appear to be selfish and in love with themselves when, in fact, their behavior is a defense to cover up how little self-love they actually have.

More Joy
A practical way to begin feeling more joy is to choose an amount of time that feels comfortable, perhaps a half hour, three times a day. From your list of things that nurture you, choose one.

Enjoy it, as Christina did watching the hummingbirds. When your allotted time has elapsed, it is fine to stop. But if you are longing to continue — go on for as long as you like. Ideally, you will find no limits to self-nurturing.

However, if you become anxious about feeling happy, it means you have hit the threshold of how happy you can be — for the moment. That is the edge you want to find, so you can examine it and gently push it back.

Even if you are anxious for a few days, that is a good sign. You are moving into new territory.

Continue taking time for your daily nurturing.

Do not suppress the anxiety. Allow it to be. By actively feeling the anxiety, instead of avoiding it, it will lessen and disappear.

Threshold to Joy
You may have only one threshold to push yourself through, but if you encounter another, edge yourself through it in the same way.

The key to breaking through the threshold is persevering, realizing your anxiety is a positive sign. You are challenging an old way of being that didn't allow for as much joy.

When you discover that it is safe to be happier, and that no one will punish you, it will become easier to be more joyful. With daily practice, you'll be able to create a life that is nurturing most of the time, rather than just during the allotted sessions.

Deepen Your Capacity for Intimacy
Often the ways we push away other people's love is the same way that we defend against the love of the transpersonal dimension. While you are opening up to feelings of oneness to benefit your physical healing, doing so will also be emotionally and spiritually healing.

By learning to experience transpersonal love, you'll also be dismantling your barriers to intimacy.

For example, during one of my workshops in New York City, a woman said, "You all are describing how relaxed you feel, but I don't feel peaceful. All I feel is the hard floor. How can I experience peace?"

I asked her, "As a child, from whom did you receive the most love?" She answered, "From my mother, but it was never safe to let in her love because it always came with strings attached. If I let it in, I felt controlled. I had to do whatever she wanted."

Peace Is Always There

I explained that the peace of the transpersonal dimension is a presence that is always there and asks nothing from us. It is like a sun that always shines. You can feel as much of its warmth as you like. I suggested that she test it, letting herself open to the peace for just a minute, to see if it had any strings.

She agreed to check it out. I guided her through the relaxation process. As she imagined her ideal place of relaxation, a favorite clearing among some evergreens, she let herself open to the experience. Her face became radiant.

After a minute, she smiled, saying, "It feels good. It has no strings. I didn't know that I could feel this way."

Each day for an hour, twice a day, as she felt the peace of the transpersonal dimension, she experienced an inner wholeness. After several weeks of daily practice, she became more grounded in universal love. She felt safe — especially when she discovered that she could control the rate at which she opened up to oneness.

Love was becoming an ever present feeling, within her and around her, that she could connect to more of the time.

Love Comes from Within

Previously, in her intimate relationships, she had found it hard to let in love from another person because of her fear of being controlled. Love felt like something that came from outside her that someone else controlled.

As a result, she had built a defense against love, the very emotion she was longing to feel, but was the most afraid to experience. While it may have been appropriate for her to defend against her mother's intrusions, her childhood defenses interfered with her adult relationships.

After three weeks of daily deepening her connection to love and letting it flow through her, she felt comfortable slowly dismantling her walls to love. More anchored in her own inner core, she felt safe being more vulnerable. As a result, she experienced a new degree of intimacy in her relationships.

Healing Co-Dependence

If you become overly needy in an intimate relationship, you'll also benefit from a similar daily practice. When some people fall in love, they become very dependent and clinging. They feel love is something that comes from outside them, from the other person.

Their way of accessing love is through loving another rather then through their own doorways that open to the infinite love of transpersonal dimension.

As a result, they feel desperate, afraid that their significant other will abandon them, taking with them their only link to love. Popular music is filled with the despair of lost love.

But when these same individuals learn to link up to transpersonal love, they feel confident in their capacity to love. Most importantly, they no longer depend on the one they love as their only gateway to love. They are connected to a renewing source of love. It feeds their souls and, in turn, all their relationships.

Ideally, as children we should have discovered that in opening to our parents' love, we opened to all love. Unfortunately, our parents may not have been grounded in the transpersonal dimension. As a result, they could not pass on this experience to us.

If you have children, you will find they will become more radiant and whole as you find ways of deepening your connection to the transpersonal dimension. Unconsciously, they will follow your example and become more grounded in oneness — in love.

Open the Door to Love

Losing oneself is another hazard of falling in love. As some open up to loving another, they involuntarily experience more of their own emotions. Feelings that were dormant, repressed in their unconscious, now become conscious. Some people are engulfed by a backlog of suppressed emotions. The experience can be frightening.

A person feels a loss of control, boundaries become blurred and the sense of self is threatened. The impulse is to run away — shut down.

Shutting down against these early rushes of seemingly overwhelming emotions, ultimately stunts our growth — emotionally and spiritually.

If you have ever lost yourself while loving another, practicing opening up to transpersonal love will help you surrender to your suppressed emotions and ride them like a wave.

Slowly opening to transpersonal love gives you a way to be embedded in something larger than yourself. Discovering how to feel comfortable in an emotional state, where your boundaries are expanded, allows you to experience your resisted emotions — and release them. With practice, you'll be able to experience them, knowing you will not be engulfed or lose control.

While you'll lose a sense of personal control, you'll experience that a deeper, wiser part of you is in control, guiding your release of repressed emotions.

Surrender to It
When you can give in to your suppressed emotions, they will sweep through you, subside and be gone.

Once you have dealt with your emotional baggage, you'll experience ever deepening textures of oneness. By accessing the transpersonal dimension at your own pace, you will be able to venture into deeper states of oneness.

Once you can control your opening up, you'll feel secure enough to give up that control — surrendering to an embrace of love — having come home.

While this process is deeply healing emotionally and spiritually, it also vastly strengthens the immune system and promotes physical health.

Afterword

To love is to receive a glimpse
of heaven.

— Karen Sunde

When I needed minor surgery to remove a small
growth on my neck, I went through the five steps
in the book.

I met several surgeons, finding one I especially
liked, Dr. Sharon Bushnell in Boston. She was glad
to use the Healing Statements since she routinely
talked to patients during surgery, telling them how
well the operation was going.

I called friends and family asking them to wrap
me in a pink Blanket of Love for the half-hour before
surgery. It was wonderful to experience their joy of
being asked.

To my amazement, I felt a lot of terror the day before outpatient surgery. It didn't make sense because it was only minor surgery. I wondered why I was so afraid.

Asked My Higher Self

When I asked my Higher Self, "What's causing my fear?", it answered, "It's not yours. It's the terror your mother felt before having major surgery years ago. You absorbed it. It is stored in your body. It is being triggered by this minor surgery."

Just knowing this, I found myself relaxing as the fear released. Naming it dissolved the terror. All these years it had been suppressed and unknown to me.

The day of surgery a good friend went with me to the New England Surgicare Center in Brookline, Massachusetts.

As I lay on the operating room table, I slipped into a very relaxed state and heard the surgeon and nurse preparing. A favorite Liszt piano concerto began to play on the radio. I listened to it instead of the music I had brought with me.

Dr. Bushnell put a cool, damp cloth over my eyes to block out the bright surgical lights and motion in the operating room. I felt a slight sting from the injection of the numbing medication.

Palpable Peace

As surgery began, a palpable peace surrounded me. Its presence was very tangible. It felt so wonderful that I didn't care how long the procedure lasted. I was absorbed in peace.

I could feel the love of different friends as their presences came and went in the room.

Then I felt my mother standing beside me. She had died years ago, but it was as if she were there, holding my right hand. Feeling surrounded by her love, I burst into tears. They were tears of joy. Her love was so strong and constant.

Once I got used to her being there and feeling her immense love surrounding me, I smiled while the surgeon did her work.

With the local anesthesia, I only felt pressure, never any discomfort during the 45-minute procedure.

When it was over, I sat up — amazed.

I was amazed by the peace and love all around me. I was amazed at my mother's presence and so grateful for the experience.

Appendix A

Vitamins that Speed Healing

by Judith J. Petry, M.D.

Need hip replacement, knee surgery or skin cancer removal? What about those nutritional supplements you give your body every day to keep it healthy? Should you stop them before surgery, continue or add more?

Chances are, your surgeon won't know what to say if you seek advice on continuing them prior to surgery. The most popular physician answer to questions about nutritional supplements is: "I can't advise you on that, it's up to you whether you take them or not."

Medications to Avoid

In the surgical setting, there are some nutritional supplements that are harmful and others that are beneficial. We all know that it's a good idea to have normal blood clotting capabilities if you are about to undergo surgery.

Your surgeon will undoubtedly warn you about taking aspirin or nonsteroidal anti-inflammatory medicines like Motrin® and Advil® prior to surgery. They affect the clotting of blood, making it more likely that you will bleed excessively during and after surgery.

Supplements to Avoid

Vitamin E, garlic, EPA (fish oil), hawthorn berry and possibly selenium also decrease your body's ability to clot normally. Vitamin E also impairs wound healing.[1,2] Studies in the laboratory and on humans have shown that normal people taking vitamin E have a decrease in the stickiness of their platelets.[3,4] This is the first phase of blood clotting. When a blood vessel is injured, chemicals are released that cause platelets to adhere or stick to the injured vessel. Vitamin E inhibits this process.

Garlic has been shown in many studies to decrease the ability of platelets to aggregate or stick to each other and form a clot to plug an injured blood vessel.[5,6] EPA, a component of fish oil, decreases the stickiness and the clumping of platelets.[7-9]

Hawthorn berry has been used as a heart tonic in folk medicine for centuries. There are only a few studies in the medical literature related to it, but they suggest that one of the effects of hawthorn berry is to decrease the clotting ability of blood.[9] The exact mechanism by which this occurs has not been clarified.

Selenium, a popular supplement used for its anti-aging and heart effects, has some anti-clotting properties, especially when taken with vitamin E.[10]

To assure you have the best chance of clotting normally during surgery and to avoid bleeding complications, unless there is a good reason to continue, **you should stop taking vitamin E, garlic, EPA, hawthorn berry and selenium supplements prior to surgery.**

You can resume most of them a few days after surgery unless you are at risk of further bleeding. As soon as your wound is healed, you can resume your usual intake of vitamin E.

Surgery aside, anyone who is taking medication that decreases blood clotting or has an abnormal bleeding condition should not be taking any of the supplements just mentioned.[11,12] The additive effect may cause excessive bleeding even without surgery.

Benefits of Vitamin A

What about the supplements that may improve your surgical outcome? There are volumes of medical literature on the beneficial effects of vitamin A on surgery.[13-15] It improves the immune system which is normally knocked down by surgery.

This is important in very sick patients with infections who require surgery. It improves wound healing, especially in people who have to take steroids for a medical condition. It improves tendon, fractured bone and intestinal healing as well.

A dosage of 25,000 IU daily should be safe for anyone who isn't pregnant. This dosage can be increased significantly under a physician's guidance in very sick surgical patients. **Pregnant women facing surgery should not take vitamin A, except under the direction of their physician, because of the potential danger to the baby.**

Bromelain Promotes Healing

Another supplement that has been shown to be beneficial for people undergoing surgery is bromelain, derived from the pineapple plant stem and fruit.[16]

The black-and-blue, frequently associated with surgery, goes away more quickly if you are taking bromelain. Another effect of bromelain is to relieve the swelling which causes some of the pain following surgery.[17,18] Bromelain can be started before surgery, and can be taken in doses of 1,000 mg per day and higher.

Vitamin C Helps Healing

Vitamin C is essential for normal wound healing. It also appears that our need for it increases after surgery.[19] Our bodies don't make vitamin C, so we require daily intake in the form of food or supplement. I recommend that patients, preparing for surgery, take vitamin C, at least one gram per day for a week prior to surgery, continuing for several weeks after their operation.

It's important to think of all nutritional supplements as medicine that may have effects of which we may not be aware.

Before you put anything into your body, read about it and talk to knowledgeable practitioners. Find out exactly what it does and what interactions it may have with other medicines or supplements you may be taking.

Dr. Petry, a plastic surgeon, was assistant professor in surgery at the University of Massachusetts Medical Center in Worcester.

Appendix B

Preparing Children for Surgery

by Peggy Huddleston

When my son, Sam, was 10, he needed a hernia operation. I realized if I were genuinely calm, he would be too. He liked the surgeon, who had a great rapport with kids and answered all my son's questions.

I told the surgeon that I would like to be in the operating room to hold my son's hand as he went under the general anesthesia. The surgeon agreed and was also glad to use the Healing Statements. Once my son knew that he would have no pain during surgery, he relaxed about the operation.

The only glitch happened just minutes before surgery. As my son sat on his father's lap outside the operating room, the surgeon began to read out loud the consent form. My son was scared hearing the things that could go wrong. I kept saying to the surgeon, "Not out loud." He finally understood and gave me the form to read and sign. To avoid this, have the form mailed to your home. This protects your child from ever hearing the information, particularly at such a vulnerable time just before surgery.

When it was time for the operation, a nurse helped me climb into a green uniform and put a surgical mask over my face. My son and I walked down the hall to the operating room with my arm around him and his around me. As we came into the room with its bright lights and stainless steel, I realized how scary the room would have been for a child without a reassuring parent. I was relieved that I could be there.

My son wanted the bubble gum flavored anesthesia given with a kid's space mask. As he became drowsy, I held his hand and felt him squeeze mine. Once he was unconscious, I slipped out of the room, joining his father and friends who had wrapped my son in a Blanket of Love for the half-hour before surgery. My son and I both felt the waves of love around us.

After an hour, the surgeon emerged to say it had been a bloodless operation and we could be with our son in the recovery room where he was still sleeping. When he finally opened his eyes, he was encircled by the love of his family.

My son was slightly nauseated and the nurse let him doze until it went away. In 1 ½ hours, he felt ready to go home. He had little discomfort because of the numbing effects of the pain medication given at the site of the incision during surgery. The next day whenever he was uncomfortable, I said, "Put your hand on the area and send it healing energy." As he did, energy flowed into his hand and soothed the area. He did this whenever he felt any discomfort. When he needed it, I gave him Tylenol® to relieve any pain. Since children recover so much faster than adults, within six days the wound had healed and he could take a bath.

One last word of advice, if your child needs to spend the night in the hospital, it's essential that you arrange to sleep in your child's room. Parents can alternate nights. Your loving presence will make all the difference in your child's experience and in your own.

Appendix C

How to Lessen the Side Effects of Chemotherapy, Radiation Therapy and Medical Procedures

by Peggy Huddleston

You have a profound ability to lessen the side effects of chemotherapy and radiation therapy using mind-body techniques. This has been documented in several research studies.[1-3] These techniques can easily be applied to reducing the stress of other medical treatments, tests or procedures.

You can diminish the side effects of chemotherapy if you:
* **Believe your treatment is a healing agent.**
* **Relax before, during and after treatments.**
* **Visualize healing imagery.**
* **Release repressed emotions.**
* **Create or find a positive support group.**

Beliefs about Chemotherapy
* **Do you welcome it — or fear it?**
* **Will it cleanse your body of all cancer?**
* **Is it healing or toxic?**
* **Do you really want it?**

You may think your beliefs don't really matter. But they do. They powerfully affect your body. Thirty percent of the people in a control group lost their hair just because they <u>thought</u> they had received chemotherapy. In fact, they only had a placebo, a a sugar pill which is a harmless substance. The *World Journal of Surgery* reported these findings.

To go through chemo more easily, find your way to wholeheartedly embrace it. You may need to ask your doctors questions that will give you the information to create a genuinely positive attitude.

Believe Your Treatment is a Healing Agent
>   * **Make it your friend.**
>   * **See it as potent healing ally.**
>   * **Imagine it sweeping your body clean.**

If you don't believe your treatment is a healing agent, <u>what do you believe?</u> Is it slightly harmful or even poisonous? Such a belief could trigger a reflex in your body which clears toxins from your system by throwing up or having diarrhea. This particular response to toxins is normal. It has been functioning in people for millions of years. If humans ate poisonous berries in the forest, throwing up removed the bad fruit from their bodies.

Although the toxic berries caused vomiting, studies show that your thoughts can cause you to throw up. Realizing this, many people have found that if they thought of their treatment as healing, nausea and diarrhea diminished or disappeared.

Relaxation
Learning to relax is another key to reducing side effects. If you are calm, you'll find it much easier to go through your treatments than if you are a nervous wreck, dreading and tensing yourself against them. Use the Relaxation CD or MP3 described in this book.

Order CD or MP3 at www.HealFaster.com or 800 726-4173. You can have them sent to you in one day by mail or email. Order form is on page 265. For an explanation of the CD and the healing benefits of relaxation, read **Step 1: Relax to Feel Peaceful.** It begins on page 31.

Once you can easily relax with the CD at home, you'll have this skill to utilize in the waiting room before your treatment. During chemo also use the CD. Once you are peaceful, you might enjoy listening to your favorite music or an audio book.

Visualize Your Healing
Towards the end of the Relaxation CD, you'll have time to imagine three end-results. For the first, imagine what you would like to say to a friend or spouse about how you felt during chemo such as:

> * **"I was so peaceful during chemo."**
> * **"Each treatment is easier."**

During your treatment, picture it healing you. For example, a man imagined that his treatment came from the healing hand of God. As a result he felt completely at peace during this therapy. A woman having chemo recalled the movie image of the pulsating finger of ET, seeing the chemo flowing from it.

Draw a picture of how the treatment will affect your body. Use colored pencils. Your drawing will reveal your conscious and unconscious beliefs about your treatment and illness. Redraw the picture until all your images are healing and the cure is more powerful than the weakened cancer.

By visualizing this drawing, you'll create an optimistic attitude which is one of the most important factors influencing how you experience chemo. Remember every thought is also a visualization.

Appendix C �* *225*

If you dutifully picture positive end-results twice a day and worry the rest of the time, your worry will cancel out the healing imagery. Instead, when fears about chemo well up, for one minute replace them with the positive imagery of your first end-result.

It's all right if a part of you doesn't believe it. Be patient. With a few days or a week of practice, you'll imagine it happening.

For your second end-result, see yourself healed. This might be a scene in which your doctor is saying, "Your test results are excellent. You are fine." Or picture yourself telling your spouse or best friend, "The doctor says I'm recovered." Use your own words to convey this idea.

For your third end-result, feel like you are totally healed and doing something you love with those you love. Put this scene as far in the future as possible. If you are 45 years old, imagine you are 65 or 75. A woman, age 45, imagined the joy of holding her first grandchild when she was 65 years old. She felt the baby's heart against her heart as she felt the joy of helping her daughter and son-in-law raise their child.

To learn more about the power of imagery, read **Step 2: Visualize Your Healing.** It begins on page 63. Your visualizations can speed your healing and alter your life. This was shown in a study at the University of Texas by Carole Holden-Lund, Ph.D., R.N. When patients relaxed and visualized their recoveries from surgery, their wounds healed faster compared to patients in the control group.

Release Repressed Emotions
Often in my work as a psychotherapist I have observed that on a conscious or unconscious level **some** people with cancer have

unresolved emotional baggage. It may cause them to feel purposeless or trapped in an impossible situation. Since these emotions suppress the immune system, it's essential to resolve unfinished emotional business.

If you have had a diagnosis of cancer, use it as a wake-up call. It can save your life if you ask, "Do I have emotions that need resolving?" If the answer is "Yes," having emotional baggage for a number of years can be a factor that depresses your immune system, allowing cancer to occur.

The solution is to contact unresolved emotions. Dive into them. Give yourself permission to experience and release them. As a result your immune system will be revitalized and can get about the job of putting cancer in remission. While "talking" therapy can help you get in touch with denied emotions, I highly recommend using one of the many types of psychotherapy or bodywork that move you into feeling your emotions.

Support Group
During the half hour before chemo, ask friends, family and prayer groups to wrap you in a Blanket of Love. Talk to them and send them an email with the exact half hour you need their love. You can **set up a free blog at www.CaringBridge.org**. Their love is a very powerful medicine for your healing. The power of positive, loving emotions to strengthen your immune system is documented in *The Biology of Belief* by Dr. Bruce Lipton, a cell biologist.

Also find an uplifting support groups because it will boost your immune system. The benefits of a support group were documented in a study by David Spiegel, M.D. at Stanford University School of Medicine in California. Women with breast cancer lived longer when they belonged to his support group and learned skills to cope with the stress of having cancer.[4]

Kathy Transforms Her Chemotherapy

Kathy called me after weathering her first session of chemo. She had gone into it emotionally unprepared, resisting the whole process. As a result her side effects were awful. She was very nauseated during the treatment. Her next dose was in four weeks and she felt very afraid of it. On the advice of a friend who had lessened her own reactions to chemo, Kathy called me.

When I explained that listening to the Relaxation CD would help her feel calm, she said, "I'd love to feel peaceful again. Ever since the diagnosis of cancer, I've been terrified." I asked her to feel the terror. It was like shock waves moving through her body. As she experienced them, instead of resisting them, they began releasing.

Although she had a good prognosis for a complete recovery, she realized she had been scaring herself to death, shocking herself with terror each time she thought of her two young children and worried that she might not live to see them grow up. While it is important not to deny these emotions, she needed to discover that she continually created them. It was a habit she wanted to stop.

Using the CD twice a day, she easily learned to relax and the exhausting cycle of fear ended. On the day of her treatment, listening to the CD before and during chemo helped her feel serene which allowed her to tolerate the chemo.

Next Kathy needed to change the way she thought about chemo, believing it was poisonous. As we talked, she remembered that she really had wanted the treatment. To see it as a healing agent, she imagined the chemo as a bright light that cleansed and blessed her body.

When we talked about the first end-result on the CD, she imagined telling her husband, "Bob, I was so relaxed during chemo today. My stomach feels fine." At home, Kathy used the CD twice a day, visualization herself feeling peaceful during treatments. When it was time for her second session of chemo, she felt in control, knowing she could use the CD to relax. During the chemo her stomach felt fine.

In between treatments, she used the CD twice a day, imagining hearing good news from her doctors about her recovery. In addition, she created days of healing. Instead of pushing herself to take care of others, she gave herself permission to do things she loved — writing poetry and playing the piano.

Love
When I asked her, "Who do you imagine when the Relaxation CD asks you to think of someone who is easy to love?" Kathy answered, "My six-year-old daughter. When I think of her, I'm filled with love." Her love for her little girl caused her heart to create a field of electromagnetic energy that surrounded her entire body. The field of energy radiated from her heart and influenced every cell, creating frequencies that are profoundly healing. Kathy's prescription for healing was to increase the amount of time she spent surrounded in love until she could live this way day after day.

Research studies from The HeartMath Institute in Boulder Creek, California show that love increases immune functioning, balances the endocrine system and enhances the cardiovascular system.

Epilogue

By reading the epilogue, **One More Way to Enhance Healing**, you'll learn how to create more peace and love in your life which enhances the biochemistry of healing.

To be inspired by stories of how others lessened the side-effects of chemotherapy, read their stories at the book's website, www.HealFaster.com.

Resources

Ways to Control Pain

In my classes I always teach "Hand Levitation," a self-hypnosis technique developed by Dr. Milton Erickson which blocks pain by putting you in a deep altered state of consciousness. People have used it during a biopsy or root channel when they could not take pain medication. Acupuncture also provides anesthesia during surgery. See page 233.

Hand Levitation

To learn the technique at home, I've made a CD which guides in using Hand Levitation. On Track 1, I explain how to use it. On Track 2, I guide you through Hand Levitation.

To master Hand Levitation, practice the technique once or twice a day for a week prior to surgery. How well it works depends on how well you master it.

When Carol Hall, a New York composer needed a breast biopsy, she wanted to master Hand Levitation to avoid pain during and after the procedure.

For a week before surgery, she practiced Hand Levitation twice a day. She called me saying, "I feel so peaceful It puts me in the same state in which I write music."

Carol had composed music for shows, including the songs and lyrics for *The Best Little Whorehouse in Texas*, one of Broadway's longest, running musicals.

As she prepared for surgery, Carol enjoyed the deep peace she experienced using Hand Levitation. Following surgery, Carol said, "I was so high from the self-hypnosis. When the nurse shook my shoulder to tell me it was over, I didn't want to open my eyes." Carol was free of any pain.

Order Hand Levitation CD

Order at www.HealFaster.com or (800) 726-4173. A CD is $19.95, plus tax and postage. You only need to use Hand Levitation if you are allergic to anesthesia.

Hypnotherapist

To find a good hypnotherapist, to release old emotions or reduce pain, see www.erickson-foundation.org. The website lists their hypnotherapists around the world.

Acupuncture

If you cannot use anesthesia or pain medication, acupuncture makes even major surgery free of pain. For 5,000 years, acupuncture has also been used for the treatment and prevention of disease. This Chinese medical system is also an excellent way to manage pain.

For practitioners contact: American Association of Acupuncture and Oriental Medicine at www.AAAOM.org

Hands-On Healing

Hands-on healing is an excellent complement to your traditional medical treatment. It works with a subtle energy that physicists can measure pulsating in and around the body.

In acupuncture, this energy is called "qi" (pronounced chee). It is directly influenced by the hair-like needles of acupuncture. It can also be manipulated by a form of Japanese massage called acupressure or shiatsu.

There are so many forms of hands-on healing that it is hard to name a few. Ask your doctor for referrals. Here are suggestions of two methods.

Therapeutic Touch

Without touching the body, practitioners use their hands to influence the field of energy that pulses in and around the physical body. More about it is described on page 126.

Two excellent books are: *Accepting Your Power to Heal* by Dolores Krieger, Ph.D., R.N. and *Therapeutic Touch: A Practical Guide* by Janet Macrae, Ph.D., R.N.

Learn it to use with your family and friends. To find a practitioner see www.therapeutic-touch.org.

Reiki

Reiki easily blends with and enhances Western medical treatments. Reiki is the Japanese word for universal energy. This hands-on healing method lets you or another channel energy into your system. It is explained in more detail on page 127.

I recommend reading *Reiki Energy Medicine* by Libby Barnett and Maggie Chambers. It is about bringing Reiki into the home, hospital and hospice. Pamela Miles has also written a good book, *Reiki: A Comprehensive Guide.*

To find a Reiki Master who can give you Reiki or to learn how to give Reiki to yourself and others, see www.ReikiAlliance.com. Have a Reiki session with several Reiki Masters. You will know first-hand which ones are best.

Ways to Release Emotions: EFT

EFT, Emotional Freedom Technique, is a form of psychological acupressure, using the energy meridians used in acupuncture. Emotions are released when you tap your fingers on acupuncture points while saying certain words. Free videos and websites on the internet show you how to use it and locate practitioners.

Feeling your emotions at a level beyond words will cause them to release and be gone. Often this causes an improvement in your health.

Many therapists encourage the release of emotions. If yours doesn't, hypnotherapy is a <u>direct</u> way to resolve emotions.

How to Handle the Bad News of a Diagnosis

Recently a client called me from the hospital, asking how to cope with a dire diagnosis she knew her doctor was about to give her. We talked about the difference between hearing the diagnosis but not accepting the verdict for her future health and healing.

Too often a doctor's opinion of how long a person might live determines how long he or she actually lives. The client prepared herself to hear the diagnosis, and used it to rally her will to live. Her doctors were amazed at her attitude that clearly influenced her recovery as the months progressed.

A dire diagnosis is also the time for a second or third opinion. On page 20, read about the book, *Second Opinion: Your Comprehensive Guide to Treatment Alternatives* by Dr. Isadore Rosenfeld.

Phone Consultation with Peggy Huddleston

For a consultation to prepare for surgery, call my office at (800) 726-4173.

You can schedule an appointment with me or one of my colleagues. The meeting can be in person or by phone.

References Cited

Your Role in the Healing Process

1. Rogers M, Reich P. Psychological intervention with surgical patients: evaluation outcome. *Advances in Psychosomatic Medicine.* 1986; 15:23–50.

2. Ackerman CJ, Turkoski B. Using guided imagery visualizations to reduce pain and anxiety. *Home Health Nurse* 2000; Sept. 18 (8): 524–530.

3. Antall GF, Kresevic D. The use of guided imagery CDs to manage pain in an elderly orthopedic population. *Orthopedic Nursing* 2004; Sept.-Oct. 23 (5): 335–340.

4. Ashton RC Jr, Whitworth GC et al. Self-hypnosis reduces anxiety following coronary artery bypass surgery. A prospective, randomized trial. *Journal of Cardiovascular Surgery.* 2000; April 41 (2): 335–6.

5. Arthur HM, Daniels C, McKelve R, Hirsh J, Rush B. Effect of a preoperative intervention on preoperative and postoperative outcomes in low-risk patients awaiting elective coronary artery bypass graft surgery. *Annals of Internal Medicine.* 2000; 133 (4): 253–262.

6. Cohen L, Parker PA et al. Presurgical stress management improves postoperative immune function in men with prostate cancer undergoing radical prostatectomy. *Psychosomatic Medicine* 2011 April; 73 (3): 218–25

7. Cowan GS Jr, Buffington CK, Cowan GS 3rd, Hathaway D. Assessment of the effects of taped cognitive behavior message on postoperative complications (therapeutic suggestions under anesthesia. *Obesity Surgery* 2001 Oct; 11 (5): 589–93

8. Gaston-Johansson F, Fall-Dickson, Nanda J, et al. The effectiveness of the comprehensive coping strategy program on clinical outcomes in breast cancer autologous bone marrow transportation. *Cancer Nursing* 2000 Aug; 23 (4): 227–285.

9. Halpin LS, Speir AM, CapoBianco P, Barnett SD. Guided imagery in cardiac surgery. *Outcomes in Management & Nursing Practice* 2002 Jul-Sep; 6 (3): 132–7.

10. Huth MM, Broome ME, Good M. Imagery reduces children's post-operative pain. *Pain* 2004 Jul; 110 (1-2): 439–48

11. Kshettry VR, Carol LF, Henly SJ, Sendelbach S, Kummer B. Complementary alternative medical therapies for heart surgery patients: feasibility, safety, and impact. *Annals of Thoracic Surgery* 2006 Jan; 81 (1) 201–205.

12. Lang EV, et al. Adjunctive non-pharmacological analgesic for invasive procedures: a randomized trial. *Lancet* 2000 April; 29; 355 (9214): 1486–1490.

13. Lengacher CA, et al. Immune responses to guided imagery during breast cancer treatment. *Biological Research for Nursing* 2008; Jan 9 (3): 205–214.

14. Montgomery GH et al. A randomized clinical trial of a brief hypnosis intervention to control side effects in breast surgery patients. *Journal of the National Cancer Institute* 2007; Sep 5; 99 (17): 1304–1312.

15.PelinoTA, Gordon DB, Engelke ZK et al. Use of nonpharmacologic interventions for pain and anxiety after total hip and total knee arthroplasty. *Orthopedic Nursing* 2005; May-Jun 24 (3): 182–90

16. Watters M, Feldman J, Schoetz D et al. The power of relaxation: a holistic approach to preoperative patient education for colorectal surgery. Abstract on page 247.

17. Toth M et al. A pilot study for arandomized, controlled trial on the effect of guided imagery in hospitalized medical patients. *The Journal of Alternative and Complementary Medicine* 2007; 13 (2): 194–197.

18. Rein G and McCraty R. 1993. The Correlation between ECG coherence, DNA and the immune system. Proc. The International Forum on New Science. Fort Collins, Colorado.

19. Rein G and McCraty R. 1993. Modulations of DNA by coherent heart frequencies. Proc. 3rd Annual Conference International Society for Study of Subtle Energy & Energy Medicine, pp. 58–62, Monterey, California.

20. McCraty R, Atkinson M, Tiller WA. 1994. New electrophysi-ological correlates of mental and emotional states via heart rate variability studies. *Alternative Therapies in Health and Medicine 1996; 2 (1): 52-65.*

21. Egbert LD, Battit GE, Turndorf H, Beecher HK. The value of the preoperative visit by an anesthetist. *Journal of the American Medical Association* 1963; 185:553–555.

22. Egbert LD, Battit GE, Welch CE, Bartlett MK. Reduction of postoperative pain by encouragement and instruction of patients. *New England Journal of Medicine* 1964; 870:825–827.

Step 1: Relax to Feel Peaceful

1. Kiecolt-Glaser J et al. Psychosocial modifiers of immunocom-petence in medical students. *Psychosomatic Medicine 1984;* 46:7–14.

2. Selye H. *Stress Without Distress* (New York: American Library, 1974).

3. Goldman K. *Angel Voices* (New York: Simon & Schuster, 1994).

4. McClelland DC. 1985 Motivation and immune function in health and disease. Paper presented at the meeting of the Society of Behavioral Medicine, March. New Orleans.

5. Rein G et al. The physiological and psychological effects of compassion and anger. *Psychosomatic Medicine* 1994; 6:171–172.

Step 2: Visualize Your Healing

1. Jasnoski ML, Kulger J. Relaxation, imagery, and neuroimmunomodulation. *New York Academy of Sciences Annuals* 1987; 496:722-30.

2. Dean D, Mihalasky J, Ostrander S, Schroeder L. *Executive ESP* (Englewood Cliffs, NJ: Prentice-Hall, 1974).

Step 3: Organize a Support Group

1. Byrd RC. Positive therapeutic effects of intercessory prayer in a coronary care population. *Southern Medical Journal* 1988; 81(7): 826–29.

2. Elsass P, et al. The psychological effects of having a contact-person from the anesthetic staff. *Acta Anaethesiol Scand* 1987; 31:584–586.

3. Kennell J, Klaus M. Continuous emotional support during labor in a United States hospital: a randomized control trial *JAMA* May 1991.

4. House JS, Robbins C, Metzner. The association of social relationships and activities with mortality. *American Journal of Epidemiology* 1982; 116:123–40.

5. Fields T. Massage therapy for infants and children. *Journal of Developmental and Behavioral Pediatrics* April 1995; 16: 105–111.

6. Bzdek V, Keller E. The effects of therapeutic touch on tension headache pain. *Nursing Research* March/April 1986.

7. Berkman L, Syme SL. Social networks, host resistance, and dents. *American Journal of Epidemiology* 1979; 109:186–204.

Step 4: Use Healing Statements

1. Furlong M. Positive suggestions presented during anaesthesia. *Memory and Awareness in Anaesthesia* (Amsterdam: Swets & Zeitlinger, 1990).

2. Steinberg ME, Hord AH, Reed B, Sebels PS. Study of the effect of intraoperative analgesia and well-being. *Memory and Awareness in Anesthesia* (Englewood Cliffs, NJ: Prentice Hall, 1993).

3. Evans C, Richardson HP. Improved recovery and reduced postoperative stay after therapeutic suggestions during general anaesthesia. *Lancet* 1988; ii: 491–492.

4. McLintock TTC, Aitken H, Downie CFA, Kenny GNC. Postoperative analgesic requirements in patients exposed to positive intraoperative suggestions. *British Medical Journal* 1990; 301:788–790.

5. Cheek DB. Surgical memory and reaction to careless conversation. *American Journal of Clinical Hypnosis* 1966; 8: 275–280.

Cheek DB. Unconscious perception of meaningful sounds during surgical anesthesia as revealed in hypnosis. *American Journal of Clinical Hypnosis 1959;* 1:101–103.

6. Wolfe LS, Millet JB. Control of postoperative pain by suggestion under general anesthesia. *American Journal of Clinical Hypnosis* 1960; 3:109–12.

7. Hutchings DD. The value of suggestion given under anesthesia: A report and evaluation of 200 cases. *American Journal of Clinical Hypnosis 1961;* 26–29.

8. Levinson BW. States of awareness during general anaesthesia. *British Journal of Anaesthesia* 1965; 544–546.

9. See note 3 above.

10. See note 4 above.

11. See note 2 above.

12. Bennett HL. Perception and memory for events during adequate general anesthesia for surgical operations. In: Pettinati HM, ed. *Hypnosis and Memory*.(New York: Guilford Press, 1988).

13. See note 1 above.

14. Bennett HL, Benson DR, Kuiken DA. Preoperative instructions for decreased bleeding during spine surgery. *Anesthesiology* 1986; 65(3A):A245.

15. Lengacher CA, Bennett MP, Gonzalez L., Gilvary D, Cox CE, Cantor A, Jacobsen PB, Yang C, Djeu J, Immune responses to Guided Imagery for breast cancer treatment. *Biological Research for Nursing* 2008 Jan; 9 (3); pages 205–14.

16. Kwekkeboom KL, Kneip J, Pearson L. A pilot study to predict success with guided imagery for cancer pain. *Pain Management. Nurs.* 2003;4(3):112–123.

17. Gruzelier JH, A review of the impact of hypnosis, relaxation, guided imagery and individual differences on aspects of immunity and health. *Stress* 2002; Jun, 5 (2): 147–163.

18. Trakhtenberg ED. The effects of Guided Imagery on the immune system: a critical review. *International Journal of Neuroscience* 2008 Jun;118 (6) pgs 839–55.

19. Disbrow EA, Bennett HL, Owings JT. Preoperative suggestion hastens the return of gastrointestinal motility. *The Western Journal of Medicine* May 1993; 158:488–453.

20. Mainord WA, Rath B, Barnett F. 1983. Anesthesia and suggestion. Paper presented at the 91st Annual Convention of the American Psychological Association, Los Angeles.

21. Rath B. The use of suggestions during general anesthesia. Unpublished doctoral dissertation, University of Louisville, 1983.

22. Landreth JE, Landreth HF. Effects of music on physiological response. *Journal of Research in Music Education* 1974; 22:4–12.

23. Burns DS. The effect of the method of guided imagery and music on the mood and life quality of cancer patients and cancer treatments. *Journal of Music Therapy* 2001; Spring, 38 (1):51–65.

24. Hanser SB, Bauer-Wu S, Kubicek L, Healy M, Manola J, Hernandez, M, & Bunnell, C. Effects of a music therapy intervention on quality of life and distress in women with metastatic breast cancer. *Journal of the Society for Integrative Oncology* 2006; 5, 14–23.

25. Evans D. The effectiveness of music as an intervention for hospital patients: A systematic review. *Journal of Advanced Nursing* 2002; 37, 8–18.

26. Madson AT, Silverman MJ. The effect of music therapy on relaxation, anxiety, pain, perception, and nausea in adult solid organ transplant patients. *Journal of Music Therapy*. 2010 Fall; 47 (3): pp.220–232.

27. Bonney HL. Music listening for intensive coronary care units. *Music Therapy* 1983; 3 (1):4–16.

28. Goldman L. Further evidence for cognitive processing under general anaesthesia. In: Rosen M, Lunn JN, eds. *Consciousness, Awareness and Pain in General Anaesthesia.* (London: Butterworths, 1987).

29. Guerra F. Awareness under general anesthesia. In: Guerra F, Aldrete JA, eds. *Emotional and Psychological Responses to Anesthesia and Surgery.* (New York: Grune & Stratton, 1980).

30. Kilstrom JF. Conscious, subconscious, unconscious: A cognitive perspective. In: Bowers KS, Meichenbaum D, eds. *The Unconscious Reconsidered.* (New York: Wiley- Interscience, 1984).

31. Kerssens C, Klein J, Bonke B. Awareness: Monitoring versus remembering what happened. *Anesthesiology,* 2003 Sep; 99 (3): 570–575.

Step 5: Meet An Anesthesiologist

1. Egbert LD, Battit GE, Turndorf H, Beecher HK. The value of the preoperative visit by an anesthetist. *Journal of the American Medical Association* 1963; 185:553–555.

2. Egbert LD, Battit GE, Welch CE, Bartlett MK. Reduction of postoperative pain by encouragement and instruction of patients. *New England Journal of Medicine* 1964; 870:825–827.

3. Huddleston MM, Bierbaum BE. Cost-effectiveness of using mind-body techniques for total knee-joint replacement. Abstract on page 249.

Appendix A: Vitamins that Speed Healing

1. J Surg Res 49(1): 98, 1990
2. Ann Surg 175(2): 235, 1972
3. Blood 73(1): 141, 1989
4. J Am Coll Nutr 10(5): 466, 1991
5. Thromb Res 44: 793, 1986
6. Atherosclerosis 30: 355, 1978
7. J Intern Med Suppl 225(731): 177, 1989
8. Ann Intern Med 107(6): 890, 1987
9. Prostagl Leukotr Essent Fatty Acids 50: 173, 1994
10. Biol Trace Elem Res 33: 79, 1992
11. Atherosclerosis 82: 247, 1990

12. Thromb Res 42(3): 303, 1986
13. Ann Surg 170(4): 633, 1969
14. SG&O 149: 658, 1979
15. Ann Surg 181: 836, 1975
16. J of Trama 5(4): 491, 1965
17. Obs and Gyn 29(2): 27, 1967
18. J Dent Med 20: 51, 1965
19. SG&O 147: 49, 1978

Appendix C: How to Lessen the Side Effects of Chemotherapy, Radiation Therapy or Medical Procedures

1. Balder L, Peretz T, Hadani PE et al. Psychological intervention in cancer patients: a randomized study. *General Hospital Psychiatry* 2001; Sep-Oct, 23 (5): 272–277

2. Eremin O, Walker MB et al. Immuno-modulatory effects of relaxation training and guided imagery in women with locally advanced breast cancer undergoing multimodality therapy: a randomized controlled trial. *Breast* 2009; Feb 18 (1): 17–25

3. Richardson J, Smith JE et al. Hypnosis for nausea and vomiting in cancer chemotherapy: a systematic review of the research evidence. *European Journal of Cancer Care* (Engl) 2007; Sep 16 (5): 402–412.

4. Spiegel D, Moore R. Imagery for cancer patients. *Oncology* 1997; Aug 11 (8): 1179–1189

The Power of Relaxation:
A Holistic Approach to
Preoperative Patient Education

Abstract

Principal Investigator: Margaret Watters, M.S., R.N., CNOR.
Co-investigators: Judith Feldman, M.D., David Schoetz, M.D., F.A.C.S.,
Mary Abrams, R.N., Cynthia Goy, R.N., Marie Catman, M.S., R.N.,
Margaret M. Huddleston, M.T.S.
The Lahey Clinic, Burlington, MA

Purpose of the Study
The psychological, physiological and spiritual effects of stress on
surgical patients are well documented in nursing and medical
literature. Most preoperative education programs focus on
cognitive and psychomotor content, overlooking the affective
domain of learning. The purpose of this study was to evaluate
outcomes for patients using a preoperative stress reduction
program, "Prepare for Surgery, Heal Faster" in conjunction with
standard preoperative education, compared to patients using only
standard preoperative education. Outcomes measured included:

1. Pre-operative calmness
2. Post-operative calmness
3. Postoperative irritability
4. Postoperative headache
5. Postoperative insomnia
6. Postoperative nightmares
7. Postoperative appetite
8. Postoperative pain
9. Use of pain medication
10. Satisfaction
11. Length of stay

Description and Methodology

Using an experimental design, a systematic random sample of 56 adult patients scheduled for major colon-rectal surgery was studied. Patients were enrolled at least one week before surgery. Experimental patients used, *Prepare for Surgery, Heal Faster*,™ a program developed by Peggy Huddleston, which included a book, Relaxation audiotape and a 1-hour telephone workshop. Data collection included three scripted telephone interviews, and retrospective chart reviews. Postoperative stress related symptoms were measured using a Likert type self-reporting scale. Descriptive statistics were used for demographic data. The Mann-Whitney U test and a 1-tailed T-test were used for length of stay and use of pain medication. ANCOVA was used to determine if differences between the two groups was due to age, which was not statistically significant.

Results

Clinically significant differences were found in all outcomes measured. Several statistically significant differences between the two groups were also found. Experimental patients were calmer preoperatively and discharged 1.6 days sooner than the control group. This resulted in a savings of approximately $3,200 per patient. Two days after discharge they had less postoperative irritability, insomnia, nightmares and loss of appetite and were using 60% less pain medication.

Perioperative Nursing Implications

Prepare for Surgery, Heal Faster™ is a cost-effective and therapeutic approach to preoperative patient education that facilitates recovery and empowers the patient as a full partner in the healing process. It has direct applications as a quality improvement initiative for both patient safety and pain management.

Cost-Effectiveness of Using
Mind-Body Techniques
for Total Knee-Joint Replacement

Margaret M. Huddleston and Benjamin E. Bierbaum

Abstract

An increasing focus on cost-containment in medical care has drawn attention to both provider and patient factors which can reduce health care utilization. Surgical procedures are costly interventions physiologically, emotionally and financially and may create significant risks of pain, discomfort and medical complications.

The purpose of this randomized controlled study of patients undergoing total knee-joint replacement was to examine by group the cost-effectiveness of Huddleston's protocol of mind-body techniques on length of stay and selected measures of anxiety prior to surgery. Huddleston's protocol consists of 1) relaxation 2) visualization 3) forming a support group and 4) use of therapeutic statements during surgery. Each of these techniques has been documented to improve surgical outcomes when implemented individually. This study investigated the benefits that accrue when the four techniques are used synergistically.

Forty-four subjects comprised the study sample. They were recruited from the New England Baptist Hospital, a Tufts University School of Medicine teaching hospital. Twenty control group subjects received traditional medical care and twenty-four intervention group subjects received a one-hour *Prepare for Surgery, Heal Faster Workshop*,™ book and relaxation audio-tape as their instruction.

Descriptive statistics revealed a significant difference in the length of stay between the two groups. The mean number of hours for the control group was 114.29 (4.75 days) and 82.75 (3.44 days) for the experimental group, Mann-Whitney U 105.5, p=0.000. In addition, using the Spielberger State Trait Inventory Scale (STAI) subjects receiving the intervention had less anxiety during the study period when compared to the control group. The mean

References ❦ *249*

anxiety (state) scores decreased over time for the experimental group and there was a significant interaction of group by time. The General Linear Model repeated measure, revealed F=5.075, p=.032. A visual analog scale to measure anxiety over the 3 time periods revealed similar significant results.

Between groups, no significant differences were found by body surface (BSA), smoking and on 11 medical conditions (stroke, MI, amputation, circulatory problem, asthma, stomach condition, depression, seizures, alcohol and drug use). No significant differences were found in the demographics using the Mann-Whitney test statistic on: marital status (married vs. other); job (working vs. not working); gender (males vs. female); age; education (HS graduate vs. not HS graduate); and income (<$20,000 vs. >$20,000).

These results are both statistically significant and clinically relevant indicating that the intervention group was discharged from the hospital one-and-a-third days (31.54-hours) sooner than the control group. Implications include the value of Huddleston's workshop, book and audio-tape as a multidimensional four-step, mind-body intervention to reduce patient anxiety prior to surgery and length of stay in the hospital.

Since clinical use of the investigated intervention reports a reduction in post-surgical nausea, lessening in use of pain medication and increase in patient satisfaction, these outcome measures will be included in future trials of the intervention.

Benjamin E. Bierbaum, MD, former Chief of Orthopedic Surgery, New England Baptist Hospital

Acknowledgments

My thanks and love to my son, Sam, Max and Napoleon for their understanding as they lived with the book while it was being written. You are always in my heart.

Finally, I thank all the seen and unseen inspirations who made this book possible. I have been deeply touched by the joyful process of writing it.

One of the joys of writing this book has been receiving so much help from friends and people who were to become friends. Their ideas always appeared just when I needed them.

Along the way the following friends read the manuscript. I would like to thank them for their advice and most of all their wholehearted encouragement: Lynne Pederson, Anne Burling, Patricia Ellsberg, Lucky Paul, Chuck Houghton, Randi Noyes, Mildred Schwartz,

Velvalee, Carman Moore, Billie Lee Mommer, Joanne Roberts, Elizabeth Hunnewell, Jane Hilles, Alexa Ayer, Wistie Miller, Bettina Peyton, Barbara Zilber, Geraldine Fox, Leigh Stewart, Nancy Claflin, Beth Shook-Blandin, Carolyn Ellis, Mary Shaw and Heather Pederson.

With a heart full of gratitude, I thank Chris Northrup for her generosity of spirit and the foreword she wrote for this book. I appreciated Judi Petri's valuable information about vitamins that speed healing.

Thanks to Merloyd Lawrence for her encouragement. I appreciated suggestions especially from anesthetist, Marcia Steinberg and anesthesiologist, Dr. Edward Lowenstein. Many thanks go to Emily Squires and Mildred Pond whose editing contributed more than they ever knew.

My heartfelt thanks to Helaine Lerner whose support has helped so many people use my book and Relaxation CD to prepare for surgery.

I am very grateful for the heartfelt support of Michelle Gendreau. Her inspired phone calls from street corners gave me good ideas. Her gifts were like Christmas presents.

Many people have given me permission to include their stories. I appreciate their trust, knowing their examples of healing will inspire others.

My gratitude is extended to Jane Chermayeff whose wondrous watercolor of Exuma graces the cover.

Over the years while living in Philadelphia, I always felt very blessed by the friendship, love and guidance of Terry Ross, Ruth and Arthur Young and Gee Elliot.

My thanks and love to my godmothers, Constance Pew High and Mary Twaddle Cromwell and my grandmothers, Peggy Dickson Friar and Roselle Woodbridge Huddilston.

I am grateful for the love, the love of books and the books written by my grandfather, Professor John Huddilston. They have inspired me.

Index

New England Baptist Hospital, 190, 249
Northrup, Dr. Christiane, ix–xii 77-78
Nurture, 205-207

Ohio State University College of Medicine, 33
Oneness, 35, 53, 199, 212
Opening Your Heart, 48–57
Operating room noise, 163
Ovarian cysts, 9, 76
Oz, Dr. Mehmet, 128

Pain, 3, 23, 65 83, 151, 161, 232
Pain medication, 3, 23, 49, 148
Parasympathetic nervous system, 14, 129
Passion, 85
Patient-controlled analgesia, 23, 208
Peace, 11, 31, 196, 208, 215
Petry, Dr. Judith, 217
Pets, 128–130
Phone Consultation, 236
Physical therapists, 71
Pink blanket of love, 111
Placebo, 89
Po, Huang, 36
Positive imagery, 63-88
Positive statements, 135–171
Prayers, 113–114, 149
Psychotherapy, 25-26
Puritan New England, 204–205

Rage, 26, 39, 76
Rath, Dr. Barry, 161
Reconstructive surgery, 160

Regional anesthesia, 136, 151
Reiki, 127, 235
Relaxation, 31-47
Relaxation CD, 4, 9, 154, 265
Releasing emotions, 25, 38, 235
Repressed emotions, 25
Resident, 17, 93
Richardson, Dr. H.P., 142
Rosenfeld, Dr. Isadore, 20

Salivary IgA, 5, 50
Sam, 221
Second opinion, 18, 168
Self-hypnosis, 94, 152
Selye, Dr. Hans, 33
Separateness, 49
Shoulder surgery, 65
Siegel, Dr. Bernie S., 143
Someone Easy to Love, 47
Soul, 199, 210
Spiritual Being, 51
State University of New York, 129
Steinberg, Marcia, 143, 163
Stress, 3, 35
Stress hormones, 14, 33
Stress-related symptoms, 4, 32
Support Person, 114
Suppressed emotions, 214
Sympathetic nervous system, 157

T-cells, 32, 33
Tao, 53
Teaching hospitals, 17
Tears, 27, 38
Tension headaches, 4, 32
Therapeutic statements, 135–171

Therapeutic Touch, 126, 234
Third end-result, 85
Thorne, Marjie, 168
Thymus, 33
Tranquilizer, 115, 155
Transfusions, 25
Transcendental dimension, 36
Transpersonal dimension,
      36, 202, 203, 202–212
Troyan, Dr. Susan, 149, 168
Trujillo, Joe, 197
Truth, 103-104
Tumor, brain, 20, 23
Tzu, Lao, 53

Unconscious, 124, 146, 167
University of California, Davis
      Medical Center, 155, 159
Urbanowski, Frank, 110
Uterus, 77, 80

"Vigilant" types, 15, 182
Visualization, 63-104
Vitamin A, 219
Vitamin C, 220
Vitamin E, 218

Wagman, Fredrica, 198
Wagoner, Dr. Peggy, 149
Wake-up call, 8
Walters, Christina, 195
Watters, Margaret, 247
Web of Life, 199
Weil, Dr. Andrew, 122
Wolfe, Dr. L. S., 139
Womb, 39
Women's Bodies,
      Women's Wisdom, xii, 78

Yin, Kuan, 52

Peggy Huddleston's
Healing Statements for Surgery

Patient's Name _____

(Give this page to your surgeon and another to your anesthesiologist. Tape a third page to your hospital gown, so it is visible as you go into surgery.)

As I am going under the anesthesia, please say:

1. "Following this operation, you will feel comfortable and you will heal very well." (Repeat 5 times.)

After saying the statements, please put on my earphones and start my CD or iPod.

Towards the end of surgery, remove my earphones. Say:

2. "Your operation has gone very well." (Repeat 5 times.)

3. "Following this operation, you will be hungry for _____. You will be thirsty and urinate easily." (Repeat 5 times.)

4. "Following this operation _____ _____."
Fill in your surgeon's recommendations for recovery. (Repeat 5 times.)

I am allergic to these anesthesias and medications:

The medications and the dosages I am taking are:

© Peggy Huddleston, *Prepare for Surgery, Heal Faster: A Guide of Mind-Body Techniques* (Cambridge, MA; Angel River Press; Fourth Edition, 2012).

Peggy Huddleston's
Healing Statements for Surgery

Patient's Name _____

(Give this page to your surgeon and another to your anesthesiologist. Tape a third page to your hospital gown, so it is visible as you go into surgery.)

As I am going under the anesthesia, please say:

1. "Following this operation, you will feel comfortable and you will heal very well." (Repeat 5 times.)

After saying the statements, please put on my earphones and start my CD or iPod.

Towards the end of surgery, remove my earphones. Say:

2. "Your operation has gone very well." (Repeat 5 times.)

3. "Following this operation, you will be hungry for _____. You will be thirsty and urinate easily." (Repeat 5 times.)

4. "Following this operation _____ _____."
Fill in your surgeon's recommendations for recovery. (Repeat 5 times.)

I am allergic to these anesthesias and medications:

The medications and the dosages I am taking are:

© Peggy Huddleston, *Prepare for Surgery, Heal Faster: A Guide of Mind-Body Techniques* (Cambridge, MA; Angel River Press; Fourth Edition, 2012).

Order: www.HealFaster.com or (800) 726-4173

40% Discount for 6 or more books & CDs

Book with 2 CDs: *Prepare for Surgery, Heal Faster*
Includes Relaxation/Healing CD and Quick Start CD
_____ copies x retail price, $29.95 _____

Book: *Prepare for Surgery, Heal Faster*
_____ copies x retail price, $14.95 _____

eBook: *Prepare for Surgery, Heal Faster*
_____ copies x retail price, $9.99 _____

Relaxation/Healing CD: English (80-min.)
Includes Relaxation/Healing CD and Quick Start CD.
_____ copies x retail price, $19.95 _____

MP3 of Relaxation/Healing CD: English (80-min.)
Includes Relaxation/Healing CD and Quick Start CD.
_____ copies x retail price, $15.95 _____

Relaxation/Healing CD: Spanish (80-min.)
Includes Relaxation/Healing CD and Quick Start CD.
_____ copies x retail price, $19.95 _____

MP3 of Relaxation/Healing CD: Spanish (80-min.)
Includes Relaxation/Healing CD and Quick Start CD.
_____ copies x retail price, $15.95 _____

**CD: How to Lose Weight: Using the Power of Your
Conscious & Unconscious Mind** by Peggy Huddleston
_____ copies x retail price, $19.95 _____

CD: Deepen Your Connection with Your Higher Self
by Peggy Huddleston
_____ copies x retail price, $19.95 _____

Shipping is an additional cost: 2-Day Priority Mail.

Quick Start CD and Relaxation/Healing CD are inside the back cover.

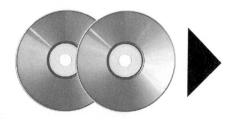

Care of the CDs

Hold the CDs with your fingertips, touching only the edges.

Fingerprints leave grease on the playable side of a CD which makes it skip. If you get fingerprints on a CD, gently wipe it with a soft cloth which is used to clean eyeglasses. Gently wipe the cloth over the playable side, wiping from the center opening of the CD to the edge. Often this will remove fingerprints, smudges and debris.

Store CDs at room temperature in separate cases to prevent scratches.

Breaking the seal on the plastic sleeve holding the CDs means they cannot be returned.

Listening to the CDs

You can listen to the CDs on a CD player and transfer them to an iPod, MP3 player or iPad.

If you need help to transfer the CDs, ask a friend. Most children who are 10 years old and older know how to transfer CDs because they have grown up with this technology.

If you Google "how to transfer CDs to an MP3 player or iPod," you will find instructions which are easy to follow.

It is best not to transfer the CDs to your cell phone. Cell phones emit electromagnetic fields (EMFs) when cell phones are turned on. Research shows these EMFs negatively affect your body and the energy fields around your body.